Art Therapy as Cumulative Trauma Repair

This book explores the effectiveness of art therapy as treatment for cumulative trauma survivors.

Bringing together case studies, research, and the author's clinical and personal experience, it outlines different clinical approaches as well as numerous art therapy interventions that are processed through somatic, metaverbal, and narrative means. It further aims to answer the question of "how art therapy works," by pairing aspects of Lusebrink's Expressive Therapies Continuum with Perry's four functional domains (from the Neurosequential Model of Therapeutics) to demonstrate how these practices may increase relational capacity and the patient's access to higher level functioning, in turn, decreasing trauma responses.

Foregrounding a person-centered and multi-dimensional approach to trauma repair and creative interventions, this book will appeal to postgraduate students in art therapy and counselling, as well as professionals and researchers in somatic work and trauma specialties.

Jennifer Albright Knash DAT, ATRL-BC, LAPT, LPCC, LPC/AODA, CCTP, RYT200

Jennifer Albright Knash is the Academic Programs Director at Southwestern College, Santa Fe, NM, USA, and an art therapist, supervisor, and counselor at Albright Art Therapy and Counseling.

Advances in Mental Health Research series

Books in this series:

Mental Wellbeing and Psychology
The Role of Art and History in Self Discovery and Creation
Sue Barker with Louise Jensen and Hamed Al Battashi

Neurolinguistic Programming in Clinical Settings
Theory and Evidence-Based Practice
Edited by Lisa de Rijk, Richard Gray, and Frank Bourke

A Study into Infant Mental Health
Drawing Together Perspectives of International Research, Theory, and Practical Intervention
Hazel G. Whitters

Film/Video-Based Therapy and Trauma
Research and Practice
Joshua L. Cohen

In-patient Mental Health Care from the Asylum System to the Present Day
A Lived Experience of Policy and Practice
Andrew Colley

Depth Psychology, Cult Survivors, and the Role of the Daimon
Oppression, Agency, and Authenticity
Linda R. Quennec

Challenging Psychiatry's Reliance on the Disease Model
A New Take on Diagnosis, Pathology and Disablement
Digby Tantam

For more information about this series, please visit: www.routledge.com

Art Therapy as Cumulative Trauma Repair

Expressive Therapies Continuum, Perry's Neurosequential Model, and Using Art Therapy Techniques to Inform Perception and Imagination

Jennifer Albright Knash

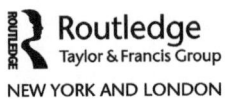

Routledge
Taylor & Francis Group

NEW YORK AND LONDON

First published 2025
by Routledge
605 Third Avenue, New York, NY 10158

and by Routledge
4 Park Square, Milton Park, Abingdon, Oxon, OX14 4RN

Routledge is an imprint of the Taylor & Francis Group, an informa business

ISBN: 9781032695259 (hbk)
ISBN: 9781032695235 (pbk)
ISBN: 9781032695228 (ebk)

DOI: 10.4324/9781032695228

Typeset in Times New Roman
by codeMantra

Contents

Figures

Part I
Laying the Groundwork

1 Introduction

The Room

I'm in a room; it's not of my own making. It was carefully constructed for me; before I moved in, it was empty and bare, identical to the room next door to mine. The matching doors open out onto a hallway. I hear no sound from the room next to me, but I know that someone is in it. The room has bars on the windows, and the inhabitant thinks that she doesn't have the key to open her door.

Over the years, I have made my room comfortable with art supplies and music, overstuffed chairs, brightly colored walls, paintings, and books filling every nook and cranny. I can see the outside and the trees; on days where I can, I open the door with my key. I peek down the hallway, and I know that I can leave these walls at any time, but the room has gotten comfortable, and though I want to explore, I simply don't have the energy. I want to go out to the garden that I've planted and pick the weeds, but I know if I start, I can't stop. Instead, I collapse onto the bean bag in the corner. It is lonely here.

I notice a stillness over time; it feels like the occupant of the other room is no longer there. I feel that she is free, free of the perfectionism and rigid rules that she had for herself that constructed her cell. Only in death could she be free from a self-imposed prison sentence that forced her into building another cell for me. I like to believe that she didn't mean to do it; I hope she didn't mean to do it. But the fact remains that she did, and it has taken many years to recognize that I was in a cell of my own and, second, to even want to leave the cell. I've tried to break free through methods that did not sustain me: years of substance addiction and disordered eating, fleeing only to be met by the terrifying arms of domestic violence and toxic systems that replicated what I was accustomed to. Chronic migraines kept me so tired that I struggled with the idea of wanting to leave. I glimpsed days without the walls around me, and on other days, I snuggled into the safety I created in an unsafe place. The walls then became of my own making; I was the only one that could make change. Other people saw things in me that I couldn't recognize, though I wanted to. Her presence made it hard before; now what was holding me back?

DOI: 10.4324/9781032695228-2

The rules—those unspoken, unwritten rules of needing to be perfect but not knowing what made something or someone perfect. And when I thought I was close, the rules would change again.

It was not until I found recovery from substances, recovery from food, and recovery from toxic relationships that I was able to open the doors and to allow myself freedom from the fight, flight, freeze, and friend responses that had plagued me for so long. There are moments where I feel the room calling, but I have the resources and the support system to resist. The journey has been winding and painful, but the rewards have been the opportunity to use my own experience, strength, and hope to inform my purpose on a path of healing and repair.

In the culture in which I was raised, therapy and getting help were not encouraged, spoken about, or even tolerated. No one grows up with the desire to be an addict, but the correlation between trauma and addiction is undeniable. I had an overactive inner critic and a high degree of perfectionism; my motivation to achieve was an asset and an Achilles' heel as is often the case for addicts. In addition, chronic migraines have been a part of my story that have also impacted many facets of my experience.

Through my own experience of recovery, working the steps, and being in a therapeutic process, I am adamant about continuing to make sure that I am as healthy as I can be so that I can support clients in their own processes. After nearly 20 years of working with women, children, and adolescents who have experienced cumulative trauma, I have found some areas of commonality that I would like to share. These findings are a culmination of my own experiences in practice, numerous trainings, and my own personal story. You will notice that rather than using the pronoun of "they," I am including myself in this text, using "we." Though there is an unavoidable power differential between therapist and client, I think it is important that the reader understands that I am part of the community of survivors in which I speak about.

A Felt Sense of the Impact of Art Therapy

I need to embody learning and to put into practice a concept to gain a felt sense of the process; this feels applicable for the therapeutic techniques that I employ. Art was an impactful and healing safety net for me from an early age, and art was the one outlet where I could express myself without others having to know what the imagery meant. It could be private or public; it could be a nonverbal act where I did not have to explain myself unless I wanted to. I could not quantify the beneficial healing power of my art process until I began my Master of Art Therapy and Counseling Degree. Working with art materials and then being able to reflect upon my work, drawing connections, and exploring metaphors allowed for repair and self-exploration on multiple levels simultaneously and implicitly. I would note that my body would either feel lighter or more energetic when experiencing symptoms of depressed mood or areas of dissociative collapse; adversely, when feeling anxious or panicked, different art materials would allow for regulation and somatic integration. At times, the story of the metaphor in the art piece was important, while at other times, the process of the creation felt enough. After being introduced to Luse-brink's Expressive Therapies Continuum, I began to understand the different areas that artmaking could reach and the levels on which it could be instrumental. Being able to research and to practice art therapy in the framework of Perry's Neurosequential Model of Therapeutics brought to light the four functional domains that will be discussed at length in the following chapters.

A Note about Self-disclosure

Carefully weighing the need for self-disclosure when writing this book, I came to a middle ground. As a supervisor, an instructor, and a practicing clinician, I have taken into consideration the questions that Bruce Moon poses: "Why am I feeling the urge to share this information…? How will my sharing be helpful…?" (2016, p. 16). When we discuss self-disclosure as mental health professionals, it is essential to look at motive and to consider whether the sharing is beneficial. Moon discusses three options: opaqueness, translucency, and transparency. I have landed on translucency, asking myself how my "artistic and relational self-disclosure will be helpful" (Moon, p. 16). It is imperative that this book feel collaborative in tone; I have found that the blank or neutral slate approach has not been useful in my own healing process nor in my work with clients who have experienced cumulative trauma. It creates a sense of coldness and judgment rather than warmth and invitation. Self-disclosure feels a bit like Goldilocks and the three bears; too much is too hot, too little is too cold (Southey, 1837). The recipe for getting it just right is tricky, but using Moon's questions as guiding principles has been useful.

References

Moon, B. L. (2016). *Art-based group therapy: Theory and practice.* Springfield, IL: Charles C. Thomas Publisher, Ltd.
Southey, R. (1837). *The story of the three bears.* London: Wright.

2 Terminology

Trauma

During the intake process with clients, we begin by discussing a bit about family systems, developmental timelines, relationship history, and levels of support, to assess risk and resiliency factors and to collaboratively create treatment planning. Clients may present with confusion and frustration, voicing, "I just don't know what's wrong with me," "I can't understand why I feel depressed or anxious, everything in my life is fine," or "Everything in my life is a mess, how did I get here?" After experiencing the history as it unfolds, we marvel together not only at the perseverance and strength that have been displayed but also at how exhausting it is to constantly persist and to appear resilient. Eventually, the body, spirit, and mind begin to tire and present as nightmares, lack of sleep, a maladaptive relationship with food, self-medication, self-harm, chronic pain/illness, relationship complications, hypervigilance and/or dissociation, fatigue, panic, etc. I have admiration and respect for the journeys of clients; however, if identity is based on being strong, at some point the human system cannot continue to operate purely out of survival. Beginning to look at strengths and adaptability is helpful; however, moving into identifying resources and safety becomes imperative to allow for rest and for recovery. We are people who have gone through an invisible war that no one else may know about, that we have possibly had to keep secret. It is heartbreaking that individuals of all ages are walking around in the world feeling unsupported and unprotected. I find that individuals who have experienced trauma are exceptionally intelligent, highly sensitive, and creative, but we have also become doubtful of own abilities and our potential to heal due to maltreatment and neglect. It is important to define trauma and to explore the impact of trauma in order to move into a discussion of healing processes.

Defining Trauma

Trauma is an experience that can alter a child's and an adult's worldview. It is something terror-filled and could result from a single incident, such as a

DOI: 10.4324/9781032695228-3

car accident or witnessing a violent event. It is important to note that what one individual might experience as traumatic, another person may find commonplace or less disturbing. According to Jaffe et al. (2005), the event itself, though traumatic in nature, is not what is most impactful; it is the person's experiencing of the event. The authors determined that there are three factors that comprise a traumatic experience: the element of surprise, lack of preparation, and helplessness to prevent the event. The American Psychiatric Association (2022) also has indicated that lack of preparation and surprise and an innate sense of helplessness are components of trauma. Jaffe et al. (2005) specified that an individual may experience trauma firsthand, may learn about the event from someone else, may be threatened or victimized repeatedly, or may be traumatized by exposure to disturbing imagery.

The effects of trauma also occur on a spectrum. Although there have been attempts to categorize the criteria to meet trauma reaction diagnoses, the behaviors and symptoms of trauma tend to be specific for each individual who has experienced traumatic events. Falasca and Caulfield (1999) identified several components that contribute to the impact of trauma: (a) the traumatic event itself, (b) the developmental stage when the event was experienced, (c) the ability to adapt, (d) the support system surrounding the individual, (e) the subject of the trauma (e.g., whether the individual observed an act of violence or was the recipient of violence, or both), and (f) the extent of the trauma (e.g., whether it was associated with an unanticipated single event, was a long-standing event, or was due to multiple acts; p. 213).

I remind my clients that there are times that the body (cell memory) remembers the trauma more vividly than the brain. For example, if there is an anniversary of a death, a traumatic event, or period of time, often an individual is left wondering what is wrong, what is causing this level of anxiety that does not have a clear source. Then there is a recall of what the link could be; the body reacts though the brain may have forgotten, leaving an individual puzzled and left to try to put the pieces together. Since many individuals are hypervigilant (fight or flight) or dissociative (freeze or fawn) at the time of the trauma, the brain may not have a clear memory or any memory of the traumatic event, but cellular memory does not forget. Memory can be like a filing cabinet; the top drawer holds easily accessible information that the brain has prioritized. The middle drawer stores items that the brain has decided to hold on to and can refer to when needed though not necessarily as readily available as the top drawer. The bottom drawer holds what the brain has basically lost, but the body is aware that it is there, resulting in a disconnect that causes a good deal of anxiety, depression, and fatigue. It is like parking your car in a large parking area while you are talking on the phone or daydreaming; when you come out of the store, there is a sense of panic initially and an ensuing frustration of not knowing where the car is. Think of doing this repetitively and continuously while still trying to hold a job, attend school, or balance family and life stressors and relationships (Figure 2.1).

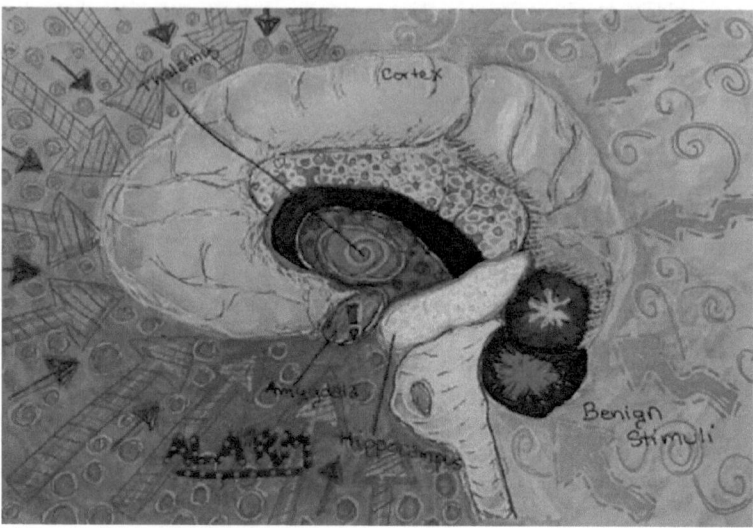

Figure 2.1 Brain art rendering. Author's rendering of the brain discerning alarm versus benign stimuli. Photograph and drawing by the author.

Van der Kolk (2014) stated that trauma tends to affect the limbic system and the brain stem. These are the parts of the brain that monitor the environment, scanning for elements that indicate either safety or danger. Van der Kolk described the amygdala as "the smoke detector" and the frontal lobes as "the watchtower," saying, "the amygdala … gets you ready to fight back or escape, even before the frontal lobes can make an assessment" (2014, p. 62). Because the brain stem is affected, there are implications for basic physiological functions, such as abnormal sleep patterns, breathing problems, urination issues, and imbalances in the chemicals in the brain and body. Higher-level functioning such as rationalization and planning, as well as decision-making and impulse control, can also be adversely impacted. In addition, a person's ability to verbalize can decrease, which contributes to dissociation and becoming shut down (van der Kolk, 2014). Simply stated, this is where the fight, flight, freeze, and friend come in. The body and the brain disconnect.

Cumulative Trauma

Cumulative or chronic trauma is a different experience. It can be more subtle. With a single incident crisis, the trauma is easier to label. When the trauma story is told, listeners immediately comprehend that something terrible has happened. However, with cumulative trauma, it is difficult to describe, to pinpoint, and the individual may not even know to call the experience a trauma as it could have been "normal" or "that's just the way it was." Individuals who have survived cumulative trauma often have not received help or have not received the correct help; often there is a misdiagnosis that leads to incorrect types of treatment since the cumulative trauma is not disclosed or is normalized.

Imagine never being hugged or comforted as a child; consider never hearing a positive phrase said to you or about you by your caregivers. Many children and adults go without basic needs being met. Unfortunately, many individuals are taught that their body does not belong to them or that they will not be protected. For adults, chronic trauma might look like long-term abuse in relationships, a toxic work environment, homelessness, abandonment, and other aspects that can be continuations of childhood experience. But if these situations are normalized by the people in one's life that are supposed to be protectors, then the likelihood that this would be disclosed in a therapeutic or medical appointment is small. These experiences are difficult to verbalize; in addition, if the caregivers are part of the therapeutic process and this process is to try to "fix bad behaviors," then the "identified patient" is highly unlikely to be forthcoming about what is happening. Instead, the "help" can feel more punitive than supportive.

Many of the adults and teens that have experienced neglect, abuse, ostracization, and marginalization as children would not developmentally have been able to comprehend that this was not their fault. It can become implanted into the psyche. This may lead to an internalizing of shame and negative phrases and self-talk that, in turn, make self-soothing, positive self-regard, and emotional regulation challenging. Self-improvement and/or self-sabotage may become a mission on a subconscious level; the goal of unattainable perfectionism can evolve into self-loathing.

Cumulative or chronic trauma has been described as a "breaking point of moral existence" (Shay, 1994, p. 164). It may be caused by an ongoing experience such as continued neglect; Perry and Szalavitz (2010) recognized the impact of neglect as a trauma category—they emphasized the long-term deprivation of a child's basic and emotional needs as a form of rupture. The impact of neglect is pervasive, altering a child's resiliency, compromising the ability to trust, and potentially damaging the child's self-concept. It shifts a person's "emotional, cognitive, behavioral, social, and physiological functioning" (Perry et al., 1996 p. 272). Shay (1994) described several factors of chronic or cumulative trauma: longer-term or reoccurring traumatic events; loss of control; hypervigilance over a period of time; a feeling of "being crazy" because memory cannot be trusted; and a persistence of betrayal, isolation, suicidality, meaninglessness, and "destruction of the capacity for democratic participation" (p. 164).

From my observations and experiences, these components ring true. There may be indications of distrust, a desire to withdraw when overwhelmed, aggression from perceived threats, anxiety, depression, attachment issues, and/or a lack of social skills. Kangaslampi, Garoff, and Peltonen (2015) also outlined the following as results of post-traumatic stress disorder (PTSD) in children: "lower verbal memory function and overall cognitive performance, impairment in academic performance, decreased quality of life, and increased suffering" (p. 128). For childhood trauma survivors, PTSD can carry "enormous economic costs associated with loss of personal income, inability to work, as well as increased utilization of treatment and support service" (Kangaslampi et al., 2015, p. 128).

One of the misconceptions in treating and addressing trauma tends to be that children and adults only need to repair or be treated for a single traumatic event. This idea is highly inaccurate in that children who are at risk for trauma typically undergo a series of traumas that result in more prolonged or sustained traumatic exposure. If a caregiver is unable to protect the child from the harm, this creates an additional layer to the trauma. Sustained exposure to trauma during childhood creates not only post-traumatic stress symptoms but also obstructions in the ability to self-regulate. Explosive anger, anxiety, inability to concentrate and to remain present, and/or isolated or violent behaviors are possible symptomology (Cloitre et al., 2009, pp. 399–400).

The PTSD criteria in the *Diagnostic and Statistical Manual of Mental Disorders*, Fifth Edition, Text Revision (DSM-5-TR) include compromises to self-concept and to adaptation to ordinary life events. Complex PTSD is composed of several traumatic incidents that may have occurred over longer periods of time. In addition, the symptomology tends to include more elements of interpersonal relationship issues as well as reactions that are more intense in nature given the sustained or repetitive exposures to trauma (American Psychiatric Association, 2022). Early on Herman (1997) viewed the PTSD diagnosis as not adequately providing criteria for individuals who have sustained long-term, repetitive traumatic events, and this critique may still be true today.

In addition, the DSM-5-TR criteria do not account for traumatic invalidation and microaggressions, intergenerational trauma, and racial trauma. These are nonlinear paradigms that are often devaluated or underestimated regarding impact on physical, emotional, and spiritual well-being. Traumatic invalidation targets anything from a person's understanding of themselves or their environment, belief systems, emotions, actions, desires, and even sensory experiences (Linehan, 2015). Types of traumatic invalidation include criticism, unequal treatment, ignoring, emotional neglect, excluding, misinterpreting, controlling, blaming, and denying reality (Harned, 2022). Hetherington discusses the concepts of "power over" versus "power-from-within" in the context of minoritized communities, focusing on LGBTQIA+ adolescents. "Power over" can be seen as "othering"—the patriarchy exerting control over a person's race, gender, sexuality, ability, age, etc., as well as in the context of microaggressions. "Power over" is linked to chronic anxiety and hypervigilance since the perceived threat is ever present due to legislation, judgment, and societal constructs (Hetherington & Luna, 2023).

In the context of intergenerational trauma, "attachment patterns that form in the context of unbearable experiences of existential uncertainty in one generation may influence the attachment patterns that emerge in the next" (Brothers, 2014, pp. 9–10). Individuals who have undergone oppression, hate crimes, socioeconomic strife, the Holocaust, bullying, abuse, etc., may experience dissociation and hypervigilance, which impact the style of attachment and caregiving. Intergenerational may also include racial trauma. Hardy defines racial trauma as

> The byproduct of persistent hyperexposure to racial oppression ... an all-consuming, crippling, and debilitating condition. ... Racial trauma is a type of unshakable hybrid of chronic and toxic stress that People of Color, regardless of other sociocultural factors, are coerced to live with.
>
> (2023, p. 83)

Individuals and communities are potentially impacted externally and internally as the oppressive behaviors begin on an external level but then can be internalized after sustained racialized abuse.

As a result of cumulative trauma (including historical, intergenerational, racialized, and/or relational trauma), intimacy and relationships understandably become much more difficult to experience and to sustain. Individuals may isolate or may be overly sociable but then exhibit a "push-pull" dynamic in relationships. There may be a tendency toward overinvestment and a desire for a much more intimate relationship than what is deemed appropriate per societally informed boundaries. Sensing that rejection may be imminent or even experiencing concern that rejection could happen, an individual may decide to either test or reject the other party. In either case, self-protection is the primary goal in either avoiding or joining into relationship, generally resulting in impaired intimacy based on the standards of perceived relational health. However, when the focus is on self-protection and self-preservation, it is reasonable that relational styles would be formulated on a basis of well-earned distrust.

Affect, Memory, and Behavior

Duration, frequency, and intensity of the trauma itself are indicators for the ways in which behaviors and symptoms will manifest for a child, adolescent, or adult. Falasca and Caulfield (1999) further divided symptoms into three categories: affect, memories, and behaviors. There can be what appear to be shutdowns or hypo arousals, in which blunt, withdrawn, or even flat affect become apparent. On the other end of the affect spectrum, individuals can become hyperactive or hypervigilant; for example, trauma survivors can behave in manipulative or overly solicitous ways to deflect what is perceived as a threat or to simply find ways to get their emotional or material needs met.

There is also a range of affect that may take place in between the two extremes (Falasca & Caulfield, 1999). These responses can reflect disinhibited or inhibited attachment patterns.

From my clinical observations and my personal experience, survivors of trauma struggle with maintaining concentration or focus, exhibited through either daydreaming or withdrawal. Conversely, there may be a display of hyperactive behaviors such as being overly talkative, disruptive, or aggressive. There may be problems in school, in the community, or at home. Behaviors can appear abnormal or disconcerting to others and sometimes echo or replicate the abusive situations themselves. For example, some people hoard food if they have previously been neglected or exposed to scarcity; others may self-harm to attempt to shift emotional pain to a more physical sensation. Depending upon an individual's ability to cope, the level of a support system, and overall resiliency, survival skills may vary on a spectrum of healthy to maladaptive. Just as there are a wide array of healthy coping strategies, there are maladaptive responses such as eating disorders, substance abuse disorders, and verbal and physical aggression. I call these survival skills that have worn out their welcome; what were once survival skills seem to turn on a person. Unfortunately, many individuals don't receive treatment for these maladaptive responses, which then may cause death, incarceration, chronic illness, and an increased potential for further trauma.

In addition to affect and behavioral symptoms, memory can be affected, resulting in intense flashbacks, night errors, and recall of the traumatic events that are uncontrollable and highly intrusive in nature. Briere and Scott (2006) discussed the fact that individuals might not remember any events or even basic information, such as where they lived at the time of the trauma, how old they were, who the perpetrator was, or other memories. Details that correlate with the timing or facts of the traumatic events might no longer be in the client's available recall. Conversely, the traumatic events could be crystal clear, including smells, colors, and details of the setting and events, but the rest of what happened during the time period may be blurry. According to Briere and Scott, these phenomena exist between two poles, the absence of memory versus the intensity and clarity of memories of a particular traumatic event; individuals can also fluctuate between the two poles. Certain smells, sounds, textures, and sights can cause a recall that feels unexplainable and uncontrollable in nature (Briere & Scott, 2006). The sensory input can elicit somatic responses (bodily reactions) that the logical brain may not have language to address.

Hypervigilance and Dissociation

Perry and Szalavitz (2010) described responses to lack of nurture and to trauma as an alternation between two states: the alarm state and the dissociative state.

In the alarm state, heart rate and blood pressure are elevated, which can appear as hyperactivity, rage, hypervigilance, and tantrums. This is the fight or flight of the stress response. The dissociative state can appear as numbness or a way of appearing "spaced out," paired with a lowering of blood pressure and heart rate. The body responds to the realization that help will not be coming, that protection is not to be expected, with surrender and collapse. Children, adolescent, and adults who have experienced cumulative trauma or neglect often navigate through the world with a dissociative and/or hypervigilant lens. People will adapt based on survival cues (Perry & Szalavitz, 2010). The following are a list of responses as outlined by Patrick Carnes (2019) in *The Betrayal Bond:*

- Sudden "real" memories (vivid, distracting)
- Extremely cautious of surroundings
- Startled more easily than others
- Distressing dreams about experiences
- Flashback episodes—acting or feeling as if the experience is happening in the present
- Distress when exposed to reminders of experiences like anniversaries, places, or symbols
- Outbursts of anger and irritability
- Distrustful of others
- Physical reactions to reminders of experiences (breaking out in cold sweat, trouble breathing, etc.)
- Recurrent and unwanted (intrusive) recollections of experiences
- Periods of sleeplessness (p. 21)

It is possible to be hypervigilant and dissociative concurrently, like hitting the gas while simultaneously pumping the brakes. This is reminiscent of a cartoon character that is running as fast as it can but is not moving; there is a paralysis and an overactivity that happen simultaneously and that are difficult to describe but unmistakable when witnessed. The person reacts with fear but cannot find adequate words or behavior to match the emotion; they reach for any behavior or affect that will assist with diminishing the panic. There is an action and a dissociation that happens with the action; self-harm is generally compartmentalized as a dissociative behavior, but when paired with hypervigilance, it seems to be somewhere in between the two states. Streeck-Fischer and van der Kolk (2000) wrote: "Chronic childhood trauma interferes with the capacity to integrate sensory, emotional and cognitive information into a cohesive whole and sets the stage for unfocused and irrelevant responses to subsequent stress" (p. 903). A child who has experienced cumulative trauma could appear to have attention deficit hyperactivity disorder or bipolar disorder symptoms and behaviors but could be struggling with emotional regulation due to a central nervous system that is simply attempting to evaluate for safety. This is true also for adults living with childhood trauma or have experienced cumulative trauma in adulthood.

When self-protection remains the primary goal, this compromises the ability of the brain to respond in a neurotypical fashion, increasing the possibility of a stress-related mental disorder. Bremner (2005) elaborated on the combination of trauma with a stress-related mental disorder that can lead to long-term changes in the hippocampus and frontal cortex, causing memory problems and ongoing abnormal fear responses as well as other psychiatric symptoms. In the long run, rather than the effects being merely psychological, there are long-lasting alterations in the brain chemistry. Given that the body and the soul need healing as well as the brain, I believe and have experienced that repair happens through creative, experiential, relational, and developmentally appropriate means.

Bottom-Up and Top-Down Processing

In many cognitively based treatment protocols, there is a propensity for the recitation of narratives and to utilizing top-down approaches, though there has been neurobiological research indicating that the storage of traumatic memories is at a somatic level. Harris stated, "Creative arts therapists overcome this paradox in trauma recovery through nonlinguistic communication" (2009, p. 94). There are marked differences between the brain's bottom-up and top-down neurological information processing when receiving traumatic stimuli. Ogden and Minton (2000) described the brain as having a hierarchy of sensorimotor, emotional, and cognitive systems. Hass-Cohen, an art therapist who studied the neurobiological characteristics of art therapy, noted that emotional arousal is seated in the amygdala, which she described as "the self's lookout"; when it detects a potentially threatening stimulus, it immediately "sounds bodily and emotional alarms" (Hass-Cohen & Carr, 2008, p. 296). When a person's amygdala becomes trained over time to perceive that a threat is ever-present, due to cumulative and/or constant exposure to trauma and chaos, the central nervous system resorts to either collapse or hyperarousal. The amygdala correlates with the brain's sensorimotor and emotional functions that produce "fight, flight, or freeze" responses (i.e., fighting off a perceived threat, running from it, or freezing in the face of it such that the body cannot respond physically or emotionally). These behaviors then become adaptive responses to relatively benign stimuli.

"Top-down" or cognitive systems regulate a person's reactions to traumatic stimuli through reason and rational thought, as opposed to the "bottom-up" dysregulated emotional arousal of the amygdala. Perry et al. (1996) described the cortex as the driver for abstract thought and language, whereas the brain stem regulates heart rate, blood pressure, and arousal states. The limbic region modulates attachment and affect, which are portions of feeling states. In addition, the authors detailed the hyperarousal and dissociative continuums that are particularly damaging to children who experience trauma and grow up with their childhood triggers to trauma intact. Hyperarousal tends to present as over-reactivity and fight or flight reactions to stress, whereas dissociative responses tend to manifest as isolation, distraction, and inattentiveness (Perry et al., 1996).

Kolb and Fantie (2009) identified a gap in the research literature between studying the structural development of a child's brain and the impact that this development had on a child's behavior and behavioral development. They delineated the development of structure-function relationships in three basic ways: (a) by correlating the structural development of the nervous system with the emergence of specific behaviors, (b) by scrutinizing behavior and then making inferences about neural maturation, and (c) by studying neural structure-function relationships in order to relate brain malfunction to behavioral disorder (Kolb & Fantie, 2009, pp. 19–20).

Piaget's systematic study of cognitive development resulted in a theory of development stages. These were organized into four stages correlating to age ranges: sensorimotor (birth–age 2), preoperational (ages 2–7), concrete operational (ages 7–11), and formal operation (age 11 and older) (Piaget, 1952). These stages are idealistic in nature; in my experience, children with proper nurturing, healthy attachment, and no exposure to traumatic events or organic brain issues may reach these stages as Piaget outlined. They are excellent benchmarks, but development may not match chronological age if there have been epigenetic factors that compromise development. Kolb and Fantie's (2009) three lenses for viewing development not only take into consideration Piaget's model but also look at both the nature and the nurture of the maturation of a child, the child's brain functioning, and the effects of that functioning on the child's behavior.

Vygotsky's (1978) social development theory emphasized social influences and their impact on an individual's maturation. The zone of proximal development describes a spectrum of learning between "what is known" and "what is unknown." The link between the two axes is the introduction of a teacher who provides guidance to assist a child in a skill that is too difficult for the child's own mastery. Vygotsky emphasized the importance of language in a child's development. Private speech is language that is internalized and assists a child in decision-making; it is a product of the child's social environment (Vygotsky, 1978). If the external speech is negative or nonexistent due to neglect, this impacts private speech and what concepts become ingrained.

The neurosequential model of development integrates social influence, developmental benchmarks, and neurobiology. Perry discussed the importance of the teacher, as discussed by Vygotsky (1978), as a resiliency factor. Having beneficial relationships with trusted adults and peers creates an intimacy barrier that protects the child. Perry factored in relational aspects versus adverse childhood experiences and the impact of these factors on the brain's development. He wrote that the brain organizes and develops in a neurosequential manner:

> The organization of higher parts of the brain depends upon input from the lower parts of the brain. If the patterns or incoming neural activity in these monoamine systems is regulated, synchronous, patterned and of "normal" intensity, the higher areas will organize in healthier ways; if the patterns are extreme, dysregulated, and asynchronous, the higher areas will organize to reflect these abnormal patterns.
>
> (Perry, 2009, p. 242)

Given that the bottom-up structures of the brain develop first, the impacts of environment and biology on these bottom-up portions will determine the health and the pattern of growth for the child's upper-level brain development.

Perry explained that the brain develops from the bottom up to ensure that infants and children have basic instincts to survive and respond on a primal level to their environments. As maturation occurs, the brain eventually becomes able to use reason and logic as well as abstract thinking. However, these areas where top-down information processing takes place are not available to infants and children. The way that they make sense of their worlds is limited to their developmentally appropriate levels. For example, they experience themselves as the center of their worlds. If their needs are not being met or if harm is being caused to them, this information can only be stored by the body and is not yet available to the mind. In addition, young people tend to view themselves as the cause of any harm or neglect (Perry, 1999).

One of the drawbacks of the sequential development of the brain is that prolonged exposure to neglect, abuse, and chaos damages the nervous system's ability to detect and discern elements of safety versus elements of danger. This results in the individual's determination that the world is entirely unsafe, which causes either an increased sensory response of hypervigilance or an overarching collapse also known as dissociation. Consequently, effective interventions that consider the impact of trauma on the body and the mind must access the "low road" functions of the brain to begin communication with the "high road" (Siegel & Hartzell, 2004). Otherwise, the trauma is merely reexperienced or discussed without repair or without regulatory skills being applied.

Because an individual's socioemotional functioning may not coincide with chronological age, it is imperative for clinicians to choose the right kind of intervention to meet the client's developmental needs. From personal observation, mood dysregulation and somatic responses are the etiology of the behaviors that are simply the external evidence of trauma. I propose that an art therapy approach be utilized to offer opportunities for regulation and repair.

References

American Psychiatric Association. (2022). *Diagnostic and statistical manual of mental disorders* (5th ed., text rev.). Washington, DC. https://doi.org/10.1176/appi.books.9780890425787

Bremner, J. D. (2005). Does stress damage the brain? *Phi Kappa Phi Forum, 85*(1), 27–29. https://doi.org/10.1016/S0006-3223(99)00009-8

Briere, J., & Scott, C. (2006). *Principles of trauma therapy: A guide to symptoms, evaluation, and treatment.* Thousand Oaks, CA: Sage.

Brothers, D. (2014). Traumatic attachments: Intergenerational trauma, dissociation, and the analytic relationship. International Journal of Self Psychology. 9:3-15.

Carnes, P. (2019). *The Betrayal Bond: Breaking free of exploitive relationships.* Deerfield Beach, FL: Health Communications, Inc.

Cloitre, M., Stolbach, B. C., Herman, J. L., van der Kolk, B., Pynoos, R., Wang, J., & Petkova, E. (2009). A developmental approach to complex PTSD: Childhood and adult cumulative trauma as predictors of symptom complexity. *Journal of Traumatic Stress, 22*(5), 399–408. https://doi.org/10.1002/jts.20444

Falasca, T., & Caulfield, T. J. (1999). Childhood trauma. *Journal of Humanistic Counseling, Education & Development, 37*(4), 212–224. https://doi.org/10.1002/j.2164-490X.1999.tb00150.x

Hardy, K.V. (2023). *Racial trauma: Clinical strategies and techniques for healing invisible wounds.* New York: Norton Professional Books.

Harned, M. S. (2022). *Treating trauma in dialectical behavior therapy: The DBT prolonged exposure protocol (DBT PE).* New York: Guilford Press.

Harris, D.A. (2009). The paradox of expressing speechless terror: Ritual liminality in the creation of arts therapies' treatment of posttraumatic distress. *The Arts in Psychotherapy, 36*(2), 94–104. https://doi.org/10.1016/j.aip.2009.01.006

Hass-Cohen, N., & Carr, R. (2008). *Art therapy and clinical neuroscience.* London: Jessica Kingsley.

Herman, J. (1997). *Trauma and recovery: The aftermath of violence—from domestic abuse to political terror.* New York: Basic Books.

Hetherington, R. & Luna. (2023). Power-from-within: Somatic art therapy with an LGBTQIA+ Teenager. *Art Therapy: Journal of the American Art Therapy Association.* 40:2, 76–83. https://doi.org/10.1080/07421656.2023.2186687

Jaffe, J., Segal, J., & Dumke, L. F. (2005). Emotional and psychological trauma: Causes, symptoms, effects, and treatment. Retrieved from https://www.helpguide.org.

Kangaslampi, S., Garoff, F., & Peltonen, K. (2015). Narrative exposure therapy for immigrant children traumatized by war: Study protocol for a randomized controlled trial of effectiveness and mechanisms of change. *BMC Psychiatry, 15,* 127–141. https://doi.org/10.1186/s12888-015-0520-z

Kolb, B., & Fantie, B. C. (2009). Development of the child's brain and behavior. In C. R. Reynolds & E. Fletcher Janzen (Eds.), *Handbook of clinical neuropsychology.* (3rd ed., pp. 19-46). Springer Science+Business Media. Boston, MA. https://doi.org/10.1007/978-0-387-78867-8-2

Linehan, M. M. (2015). *DBT skills training manual* (2nd ed.). New York: The Guilford Press.

Ogden, P., & Minton, K. (2000). Sensorimotor psychotherapy: One method for processing traumatic memory. *Traumatology, 6*(3), 149–173. https://psycnet.apa.org/doi/10.1177/153476560000600302

Perry, B. D. (2009). Examining child maltreatment through a neurodevelopment lens: Clinical applications of the Neurosequential Model of Therapeutics. *Journal of Loss and Trauma, 14,* 240–255. https://psycnet.apa.org/doi/10.1080/15325020903004350

Perry, B. D., Pollard, R., Blakly, T., Baker, W., & Vigilante, D. (1996). Childhood trauma, the neurobiology of adaptation, and "use-dependent" development of the brain: How "states" become "traits." *Infant Mental Health Journal, 16*(4), 271–291.

Perry, B. D., & Szalavitz, M. (2010). *Born for love: Why empathy is essential—and endangered.* New York: William Morrow.

Piaget, J. (1952). *The origins of intelligence in children.* New York: International Universities Press.

Shay, J. (1994). *Achilles in Vietnam.* New York: Scribner.

Siegel, D., & Hartzell, M. (2004). *Parenting from the inside out.* New York: Penguin.

Streeck-Fischer, A., & van der Kolk, B. A. (2000). Down will come baby, cradle and all: Diagnostic and therapeutic implications of chronic trauma on child development. *Australian and New Zealand Journal of Psychiatry, 34,* 903–918.

van der Kolk, B. (2014). *The body keeps the score: Brain, mind, and body in the healing of trauma.* New York: Viking Press.

Vygotsky, L. S. (1978). *Mind in society: The development of higher psychological processes.* Cambridge, MA: Harvard University Press.

3 Connecting the Expressive Therapies Continuum (ETC) and the Four Functional Domains (from NMT)

When I moved into internship and ultimately into being an art therapist and counselor, I found that meeting with clients felt like what I had been training for my whole life. Sitting with another human and being able to share their energy, sense their pain and their joy, but more importantly, sense their own inner way of knowing and healing themselves were a profound experience. Recognizing this and recognizing the power of art therapy in the healing process, it became imperative to be able to frame these experiences in terminology that would also translate to conversations with medical professionals, caregivers, and clients themselves. When I started the doctorate process and my research, I wanted to put the pieces together, to work backward essentially to understand why the way I worked intuitively seemed to be having a positive impact on individuals with cumulative trauma. At the time I started practicing, art therapy and the link to neurobiology seemed to be in its infancy. It felt impossible at times to label and to construct explanations for something that had been innate and instinctual. I was familiar with the Expressive Therapies Continuum (ETC) but unfamiliar with Perry's four functional domains. My only exposure had been to the Adverse Childhood Experiences (ACEs) literature and the long-term impact of traumatic events (Anda et al., 2006). After becoming familiar with the Neurosequential Model of Therapeutics (NMT) and the four functional domains, the pieces of the puzzle clicked into place.

When considering media, interventions, treatment planning, and modalities of therapy, operating within the frameworks of the ETC and the NMT in tandem will allow for decreased client and therapist frustration as well as increased satisfaction and participation in the therapeutic process/strengthening of the therapeutic alliance. Within the NMT, there is a linear progression which indicates the need to integrate the sensory elements and to regulate emotions to improve relational capacity and to engage in cognitive, higher-level executive functioning. This mirrors the process in the ETC as symbolic and cognitive levels are difficult to engage if the other levels have not been incorporated. One benefit of art therapy is the ability to utilize all functional domains and levels of the ETC in tandem. "The ETC is lateralized (not polarized) with differing depths to declarative left hemisphere and

DOI: 10.4324/9781032695228-4

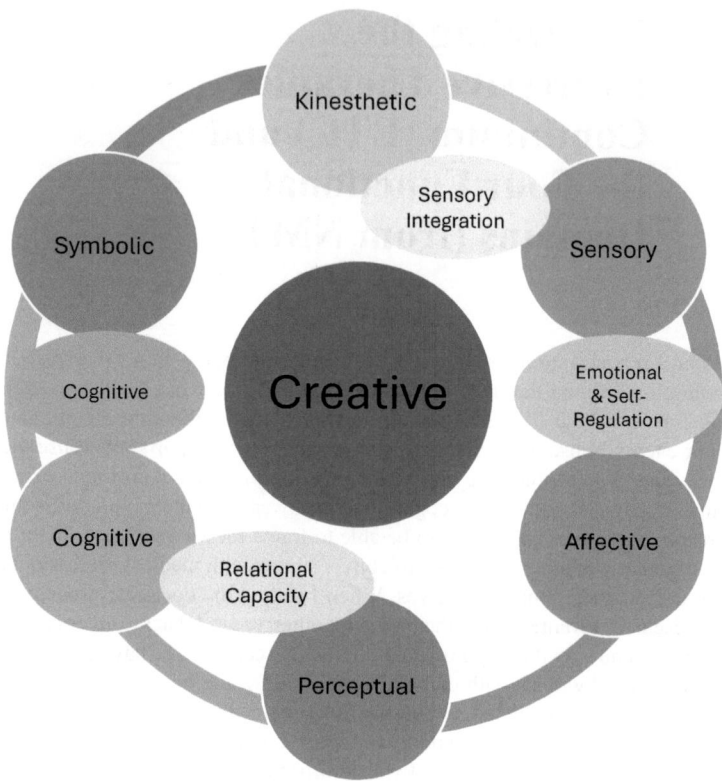

Figure 3.1 Chart depicting the interconnection between the levels of the ETC and the NMT four functional domains.

non-declarative right hemisphere processing. Movement in artmaking can go in multi-directions on the continuum in a single art process" (Kolodny, 2021, p. 116). It is ideal to move into a creative or flow state where an individual is fully grounded and resourced somatically to increase connection and to enhance metaphorical/symbolic language. This provides a bridge between bottom-up and top-down processing (Figure 3.1).

Sensory Integration and the Kinesthetic/Sensory Level

The kinesthetic/sensory Level engages areas of the brain that are connected to preverbal functioning; this level is all about rhythmic movement, an appeal to the five senses, and exploration. The sensory level of the ETC focuses attention on the sensory exploration of art media, surfaces, and textures. The kinesthetic level of the ETC is comprised of repetitive movements that can be regulatory or expressive in nature. Sensory integration entails building tolerance and ability to engage in somatosensory activities that appeal to and utilize the five senses. For example, a client selects model magic at the beginning of the session. They begin by first trying to unwrap the media (for some reason this is always somewhat impossible) where the therapist helps by cutting the wrapper. The experience of this and how the clay substance sticks somewhat to the wrapper is an introduction of partnership in the process; the client hears the wrapper crackle, smells the model magic, notes the color, and tests the texture on their hands. Though uncertain, they proceed, perhaps tentatively or possibly diving into movement with the media and verbalizing these sensations and experiences.

With immersion into the kinesthetic level, the movement can be picking at pieces of the clay in a rhythmic fashion, rolling the clay with pressure with the hands and making a snake shape, pounding the clay with the fists, or slapping the clay with an open palm. In any regard, the hope is that the somatic response will create an increased tolerance and eventual appeal to the sensory experiences. The kinesthetic and the sensory levels lie on a horizontal continuum; they are not mutually exclusive, but the kinesthetic may preclude the sensory and vice versa. Lusebrink offers that there are moments of overshadowing where the kinesthetic can present as aggressive movement that is unproductive or destructive and/or the opposing absorption in the sensory component to the point that movement is unavailable (Lusebrink, 2010). This appears as being either in the collapsed or dissociative state below the optimal arousal zone of the window of tolerance or in the hyper-aroused state above the optimal arousal zone. When this occurs, working on regulation is essential; it can also be difficult to discern if a series of movements are productive or unproductive. Offering different options of materials that are less fluid can be helpful (colored pencils, markers, crayons) or even doing a check in with the body to notice areas of overwhelm or underwhelm and offering regulatory movements/breathing.

For the sensory integration aspect, if the tolerance is increased, this may allow for the introduction of new experiences and the widening of curiosity to explore options in the creative realm, the therapeutic realm, and potentially a generalization to a client's world. Perry offers the concept of "dosing" with therapeutic interventions; offering sensory integrative experiences in repetitive intervals throughout the day and the week can be essential in order to create new opportunities for development and "rewiring" of the brain. This is where offering training to caregivers as well as educators and creating options for all involved in a client's life is necessary for reparative experiences. Consider a physical therapy experience where multiple exercises are assigned for different times throughout the day in between appointments; this strengthens the afflicted area on a physical level. Given that cumulative trauma (with an emphasis on neglect or repeated childhood abuse) impacts the way the brain receives sensory input,

> The principle of use dependence is at the heart of effective therapy. Therapy seeks to change the brain. Any efforts to change the brain or systems in the brain must provide experiences that can create patterned, repetitive activation in the neural systems that mediate the function=dysfunction that is the target of therapy.
>
> (Perry, 2009, p. 244,)

Emotional and Self-Regulation and the Perceptual/ Affective Level

Emotional regulation is a constant "sweet spot" in the therapeutic milieu; if a client and therapist both operate from an emotionally regulated state, this allows for more integration of information and emotion since the autonomic nervous system is responding from the optimal arousal zone/window of tolerance. When the self is regulated, there is a stabilization of emotions and a decrease of hypervigilance and/or dissociation; the somatic self is not responding in fight, flight, freeze fashion. There is a greater correlation to safety. The ability to self-soothe and to be soothed is more accessible.

In the perceptual/affective level of the ETC, there is an awareness of form in the artwork as well as an awareness of appropriate affect. In the perceptual, language joins the previous nonverbal expression, but this is the language of colors, lines, and shapes. "The P component appears to reflect an emphasis on the processes of the ventral stream of visual information processing with its emphasis on differentiation and clarification of forms and shapes" (Lusebrink, 2010, p. 171). The affective is the emotional involvement to this process. Increased color and variety as well as the value of color become more prevalent. If the affective becomes overarching, the emotions may take over the process resulting in lack of formation or disorganization in the artwork. The perceptual could also dominate, blocking the emotional expression and resulting in a compulsivity in form creation or lack of attention to form. The affective component relies heavily on the amygdala's emotional processing.

Self-regulation and emotional regulation are not involuntary states of being, especially for individuals who have experienced cumulative trauma. This is a constant area of intentional practice; in order for the perceptual and affective levels to be somewhat balanced and accessible, self-regulation is essential. There is a tendency to move into the "treatment phase" for anxiety and symptoms of traumatic stress, venturing prematurely into the cognitive realm, asking that a client be able to complete a worksheet or a brain-based intervention that neglects the involvement of the body and the somatic responses. This is where somatic and art-based interventions can quickly offer an element of regulation and can be "prescribed" for home, work, and school usages.

Returning to the example of working with model magic, when somatic and emotional regulation is accessible, the rolling of the model magic may slow down, taking a more intentional turn to the movement. A creature with spots may begin to take shape; the client might note sadness or happiness in themselves as the creature emerges. There is an awareness of the both the imagery coming forward and the emotional state of the creator. The artmaking may be soothing or may be emotionally evocative, but when this phase is at its optimal state, the creator is feeling regulated and feeling at home in themselves and with their emotions whether pleasant or unpleasant. They are in the optimal arousal zone of the window of tolerance, which creates a solid foundation for an exploration of relational capacity and a foray into the cognitive.

Relational Capacity and the Cognitive/Symbolic Level

The cognitive level of the ETC allows for generalization of concrete experiences. This is where decision-making and problem-solving become available and utilized. The symbolic level allows for symbolism and personal metaphor, "an immersion in a symbolic mode of thought, and the perception of self and others in a symbolic context" (Lusebrink & Hinz, 2020). As opposed to the previous levels of the ETC and the NMT, bottom-up processes have been integrated, and now top-down art therapy and cognitive experiences have been engaged.

Increasing relational capacity is key for this next step with creative and experiential elements to be accessible. Once sensory integration and emotional regulation have been practiced and strengthened (use dependent), then relational capacity can be expanded to allow for a foray into the cognitive level. This is where a true therapeutic alliance can be conceived, and then the safety in the alliance allows for the "top-down" influences of the prefrontal cortex. The quality and quantity of healthy human interactions versus those that are abuse or unhealthy are important to weight; relationships that are healthy and constant are essential resiliency factors. Being able to create a therapeutic alliance is impossible when relational capacity is not expanded or available; for intersubjective experiences to take place in the therapeutic milieu, safety in the forms of emotional regulation and sensory integration must be accomplished. Though it is easiest to discuss these aspects of the ETC and NMT in linear levels, they are in fact more circular and rhythmic, often needing repetition and possibly repair.

To return to the model magic creature, at this point on the ETC and the NMT, an individual can now tell a story about their creature. The creature may now have a name and may also possess characteristics that are like its creator, the storyteller. For example, an adolescent I worked with talked about the snake they created in the context of an abusive adult, describing the actions of the adult in correlation to the behaviors of the snake. The client then adjusted the story, stating that they felt that they were the snake, adding a rattle to the tail of the snake. The client voiced that when they were afraid, they tried to warn people that they were about to strike but that often they didn't feel that people recognized how their actions were impacting the stress response of the client. The client and I brainstormed ideas of how to make the snake feel safer and created these elements in the snake's environment out of clay, engaging in problem-solving. In addition, the client was able to name the feelings that the snake was having, especially fear which was not acceptable to display for the client; anger and self-protection were acceptable to display but fear connoted vulnerability. Being able to vacillate between an externalization of qualities (the snake as an abusive adult) to self-awareness and self-reflection (the snake as a symbol of the client's fear) appeared to be a result of a sense of trust within the therapeutic alliance.

Creative and Cognitive Functioning

Gotlieb et al. (2019) posited that:

> Imagination is the seed that may ultimately produce the rare fruit of creativity. If this is so, it is also the case that cultural context is the wind and angle of the sunlight affecting the direction in which the imagination tree grows. Environmental support for creativity and personality traits (e.g., openness to experiences) are the fertile soil that determines the extent to which the tree has the needed nutrient to grow. The default mode network and other networks in the brain are the xylem and phloem tissue setting biological constraints on how the tree produces fruit.
>
> (p. 723)

This quotation is an excellent summary of imagination and what it takes for imagination to be cultivated and nourished. For individuals living in fight, flight, and freeze, moving into states of imagination and the creative level of the ETC may be difficult. We are not open to new experiences and feeling nourished to grow when we are in survival mode. Being in the optimal arousal zone and having moved within the four functional domains to the cognitive and being in the creative realm of the ETC, then imagination can be employed more freely and more fluidly. The creative and cognitive levels are not a final destination but hopefully an integral and often visited stop in the therapeutic journey, which again is more cyclical in nature. There may be times of creativity and cognition that then become interrupted by an external or internal trigger; this is why creating safety in the therapeutic alliance is key to navigate these moments and to offer resourcing to return to regulation.

References

Anda, R. F., Felitti, V. J.,Bremner, J. D., *et al.* (2006). The enduring effects of abuse and related adverse experiences in childhood. *European Archives of Psychiatry and Clinical Neuroscience, 256,* 174–186. https://doi.org/10.1007/s00406-005-0624-4

Gotlieb, R., Hyde, E., Immordino-Yang, M., & Kaufman, S. (2019). Imagination is the seed of creativity. In J. Kaufman & R. Sternberg (Eds.), *The Cambridge handbook of creativity* (Cambridge Handbooks in Psychology, pp. 709–731). Cambridge: Cambridge University Press. https://doi.org/10.1017/9781316979839.036

Kolodny, P. (2021). Healing addiction and trauma with the expressive therapies continuum and a neurosequential art approach. In P. Quinn (Ed.), *Art therapy in the treatment of addiction and trauma* (pp. 115–134). London: Jessica Kingsley Publishers.

Lusebrink, V. B. (2010). Assessment and therapeutic application of the expressive therapies continuum: implications for brain structures and functions. *Art Therapy: Journal of the American Art Therapy Association, 27*(4), 168–177. https://doi.org/10.1080/07421656.2010.10129380

Lusebrink, V. B., & Hinz, L. (2020). Cognitive and symbolic aspects of art therapy and similarities with large scale brain networks. *Art Therapy: Journal of the American Art Therapy Association, 37*(3), 113–122. https://doi.org/10.1080/07421656.2019.1691869

Perry, B.D. (2009). Examining child maltreatment through a neurodevelopmental lens: Clinical applications of the Neurosequential Model of Therapeutics. Journal of Loss and Trauma, 14:4, 240–255, DOI: 10.1080/15325020903004350

Part II
Exploration of Art Therapy Approaches

4 Directive versus Nondirective

So many of the choices that I make as an art therapist feel intuitive, but then as I write this chapter, I recognize the importance of taking a step back to examine the benefits and the constraints of the options available in a session. There is value to structure and specificity provided by offering a directive or a couple of directive options as well as allowing for greater choice and collaboration by simply furnishing media (an art supply buffet so to speak). Depending on the order of the session (is it the first, the second, the twentieth?), the goal of the session, what the client's emphasis is for the day, the treatment plan trajectory, etc., this helps determine and narrow the options of a more structured or a less structured approach. I am cognizant that being flexible and adaptive to the client's needs is more important than any plan. I have purchased or sourced the "perfect" material for a directive for an individual or a group to then have the focus of the session shift entirely due to events of a past week. Being able to let go of my intentions to best serve the needs of the client is essential; we inherently know what is healing, but cumulative trauma might separate us from this knowledge until it is reawakened in our somatic experiences. Adapting a plan to fit the needs of a client allows for collaboration and democracy in session as opposed to "the therapist knows best." The client knows what their body needs inherently; it is the art therapist's role to help a client reconnect to this implicit knowledge and to reacquaint themselves with their own bodies' healing abilities.

Directive Purposes and Benefits/Constraints

Keeping cultural considerations, developmental stages, and trauma history at the forefront throughout the therapeutic process is essential. This can be challenging if the client has not disclosed or cannot recall key aspects of memory that could be jarring; having a safe container allows for a cushion for moments such as these. When choosing an intervention, assessment, or directive, there will be aspects of a person's history or cultural constellation that may be in a shadow area for yourself and/or for the client. Working slowly and deliberately is key.

DOI: 10.4324/9781032695228-6

The directive process can offer more specific information and can also provide structure that might feel less daunting at the beginning of working with a client. It can also provide direction for treatment planning, diagnosis, and overall levels of functioning. I tend to stay away from simply information gathering, which can feel voyeuristic, prying, and like an archeological expedition. I choose a directive based on several factors:

1   What is the directive or assessment created to address? Does it adapt or fit this situation or intention?
2   How will this be helpful for the client and for the therapeutic trajectory?
3   What is the level of healing or repair benefit?
4   What is the potential risk?

Offering art supplies to a new client without direction can feel overwhelming given the amount of choice as well as perhaps a lack of familiarity with the materials themselves. For individuals who don't have an art background or positive experiences perhaps in art classes (or even the opportunity to have an art class), this can elicit a fear response that will throw a roadblock into the therapeutic process. If a directive approach feels overly structured without the options of choice, this can feel authoritative and overbearing, stymieing the creative process or potential for flow. For minoritized individuals, coming into too much ambiguity or a situation without choice or options could potentially cause rupture in possible relationship building. Directive interventions and/or assessments can engage many levels of the four functional domains and the Expressive Therapies Continuum, which is a benefit. What I also find is that being able to assess potential for post-traumatic growth/stage of change is useful; if I'm operating out of an idea of where I think the client is versus where they really are, there can be unnecessary tension.

There are more open-ended directives versus those with more focus; offering a choice perhaps between two or three media options can expand the effectiveness of a directive. For example, asking a client draw, paint, or sculpt how they feel this week if the emotion(s) jumped out of their body and landed on the page or the table is fairly fluid and open. This offers opportunity for sensory integration and regulation; it could unlock a story about the week or metaphor exploration, which would connect the bottom-up process to the top-down one. For a more structured task, asking a client to utilize markers or colored pencils (less fluid materials) and to complete the Bridge Drawing (Hays & Lyons, 1981) would be more concrete with more defined media choice. The directive of the Bridge Drawing is to draw a picture of a bridge going from someplace to someplace, indicating where you are in the picture and drawing the direction of travel. However, I tend to customize this drawing process more to the client. I will ask the client to draw a bridge and put themselves somewhere in the picture, omitting the directionality. This opens a discussion of the possibility of going in multiple directions, potentially depicting themselves as a symbol in the image (the sun, the water, a fish, a bird, in a car, etc.). It also allows for discussion of past, present, and future as well as where the client may currently be versus where they possibly would like to be. We can utilize this information for goal-setting and for a consideration of action steps. The emotions art directive and the Bridge Drawing both have merit; their purposes and sensory/regulatory potential are different. The emotions art directive offers fluidity and openness; the Bridge Drawing might offer more information about where a client is in the treatment process or with a specific issue.

I had a client tell me that one of her favorite interventions we had done was a collage about her preferences; she used two sheets of paper where she chose magazine pictures of appealing images versus less appealing imagery. She stated that she had forgotten what she cared about and used to do for leisure activities. She started a collage journal at home, which she then started bringing in weekly (without being prompted by me) to share her feelings from the week. This gave her a way to communicate and to track her emotional patterns, offered a window into her broader life, and created a starting point each session to process and to explore. She was able to recognize stressors and positive stimuli in her life; we talked about how to cope with the stressors and ways to augment and to expand upon the positive stimuli.

Adversely, I have had the experience of offering a directive that fully fell flat or increased arousal; this offered an opportunity to brainstorm with the client to consider other options. I think even the most experienced or well-intentioned art therapist has had this occur as there are things that lie in a client's unconscious that may not present itself until the art process begins. This is where increased choice and transparency can decrease adverse impact. Practicing informed consent about the advantages and potential risk regarding an intervention is important when trust and rapport building are in their infancy.

The Nondirected Art Process

I find that after working with a client for some time and having cultivated a therapeutic relationship, we can move away from more directive options and instead delve into greater media choice to enhance repair. We are no longer in the initial treatment planning or assessment stage; we are journeying into areas of imagination, creativity, autonomy, and self-direction. There is more comfortability for the client. This is when I offer media and I might offer loose ideas, but then the individual can create their own art pieces without as much of my influence. We have entered a place of greater self-trust for the client and a tapping into imagination and creativity that might not have been accessible before; this is something that must be honed and experienced in a safe and secure forum. This is also the space where the four functional domains and the ETC are especially important to be mindful of.

I have an adolescent client who tells me where her mood is, what type of week she has had, and what she is needing from me through the media she chooses that week. If she selects beads and jewelry making, I know that she is feeling creative but is wanting sensory integration and emotional regulation. She tends to make jewelry for friends and tells stories as she works with the beads, divulging more about these relationships. If she chooses a box, this is most often for herself; on these days, she talks more in depth about her body and safety. Coloring page days are usually at a lowest point for the client and safety planning may be necessary; I say this because these are times when creative energy is too hard to access, and she is desiring the least taxing and the most regulating option. She has voiced only wanting to have to choose colors and considering the next right indicated step. Her body knows what she needs; I am there to give her the tools and to support her in her process. I am grateful for the rapport we have built, for the permission she has given me to be present for her.

References

Hays, R. E., & Lyons, S. J. (1981). The bridge drawing: A projective technique for assessment in art therapy. *The Arts in Psychotherapy, 8*(3–4), 207–217. https://psycnet. apa.org/doi/10.1016/0197-4556(81)90033-2

5 Collaborative Approach to Media and/or Directives

"Welcome to the paint, welcome to the paper, welcome to deep self-expression, welcome to this safe place for your story" (Schroder, 2004, p. 71). This quote from Schroder offers a proverbial welcome mat to the art therapy space, whatever that might look like. As art therapists, the dream is often to have a beautiful, clean, organized space full of a variety of supplies; sometimes this dream is not applicable or achievable depending on your role or setting. When I first started, I was working in therapeutic foster care, going from home to home, doctor's offices, school, courthouses, or restaurant parking lots. My office was a milk crate in my trunk and a messenger bag full of Uno cards, crayons, markers, colored pencils, construction paper, tempera or watercolor paint, and model magic. Though I was unaware at the time, I was able to offer a full range of materials based on the Expressive Therapies Continuum and the four functional domains. The youth I worked with referred to this as "the magic bag" and enjoyed a good rummage to find what they wanted to use for the time we had together. There were moments of deep connection and repair in my car or in a waiting room; this was later applied to many agency settings where some art materials were unsafe due to the level of care. Rather than feeling limited, it was an excellent time to become creative in partnership with clients. For example, not having scissors was an opportunity for somatic regulation, for emotional expression, and for problem-solving by ripping, folding, and having visceral moments with collage materials. This opened conversations about what it would look like to feel safe enough with yourself to have scissors again or to engage in self-trust.

Moon (2003) wrote,

> We make art in order to responsively interact with clients. We make art in order to engage in a kind of spiritual practice and to participate in soul-making. Finally, we make art in order to form authentic relationships with others and with ourselves.
>
> (p. 19)

DOI: 10.4324/9781032695228-7

When a client first comes into the office, I hope that it doesn't look like an office. I have the luxury of being able to control the environment (much more so than in many of my past roles as a clinician). I offer people a "tour," familiarizing them with where everything lives. I want them to know that they are welcome and that they have access to any of the art supplies, games, sand tray, and other options that are available. We discuss comfort with art materials; we discuss whether an "idea or an inspiration" is needed or if there is an idea bubbling. We might begin with a scribble drawing or a direction toward a specific media. When I begin with artmaking in session, I will often make art alongside, to engage in a collaborative process. There are exceptions; if an individual needs a therapeutic "third hand" with an art process, I will offer this rather than working on a piece of art myself. When we get to a place of processing artwork, I will either put the art I'm working on to the side or I will offer it as a reflection to what the client has been working on. I choose either to create something in a journal process I have that is ongoing or another option that does not require my full focus so that I can be present for the client's needs while still engaging in artmaking with the client. I appreciate the opportunity for our artmaking to create intersubjective space where connection and repair can occur.

If clients have materials that they have from home or projects that they are working on independently that they would like to bring into the therapeutic space, I welcome this. In addition, if we begin a process in session that can be continued at home, I love this. Creating a bridge between the therapeutic world and the outside world helps generalize skills and progress into other areas of a client's life. I have clients who like working on tablets in digital media and utilize this strategy between or in sessions.

Something to keep in mind is that art materials can be restrictive in cost; this is where ingenuity and partnership with clients can be helpful. Working with found objects, recycled materials, and natural elements can be cost-effective and widen accessibility for clients to create art at home outside of session. This can be culturally responsive and/or interact with an already existing cultural and/or communal practice. When clients begin taking projects home with them to work on, begin a creative journal process, start crocheting, making digital art, etc., this is an indication that our journey is moving past our time together and generalizing into self-propelled regulatory and healing opportunities. I encourage art therapy work at home in between sessions; Bruce Perry talks about therapeutic moments as a "dosing process" where regulatory practices are offered several times per day in small amounts. In recovery and in neuropsychology, there is the concept that it takes 90 days to build a new neural pathway in the brain. I found this to be true on a personal level, and I've seen evidence of this with clients. If we can work together to create repetitive, healing opportunities that are imaginative forays into self-exploration and self-reflection, substantial change and repair can occur.

References

Moon, B. L. (2003). *Essentials of art therapy education and practice.* Springfield, IL: Charles C. Thomas Publisher, Ltd.

Schroder, D. (2004). *Little windows into art therapy: Small openings for beginning art therapists.* Philadelphia, PA: Jessica Kingsley Publishers.

Part III

Integration and Regulation

6 Engaging Sensory Integration and the Kinesthetic/Sensory Levels of the Expressive Therapies Continuum

Cornelia Elbrecht (2018) discusses sensory awareness and body perception; sensory awareness is a "felt sense" and focuses primarily on the activation of sensations in the body and in the environment, eliciting general responses of a sensation being positive or negative. Body perception is a greater introspective process of connecting to the actual parts of the body and ways to decrease, alter, or increase sensation to alleviate pain. Beginning with the bottom-up approach is essential to increase sensory awareness and ultimately sensory engagement and integration. Once sensory awareness and integration are available, emotional and self-regulation are more readily available, which can parallel body perception that Elbrecht references. Sensory experiences, whether positive or negative, must first come into an individual's awareness and processed/categorized as "tools in the toolbox" or rejected as unpleasant or potentially triggering. Once identified, they can become part of regulatory processes or experiences.

The kinesthetic/sensory level of the ETC can be utilized to make these identifications and classifications of positive or negative to activate sensory awareness. There are several materials that I find most beneficial to introduce during this level and to create sensory experiences that are hopefully inviting and playful. Scented markers and essential oils are good forays into olfactory awareness; it is important to ask about scents as potential triggers for health issues (migraines, seizures, etc.) or possible associations to traumatic events prior to bringing in smells.

Determining favorite colors and textures is helpful given that likes and dislikes can be forgotten in the wake of cumulative trauma and possible dissociation and separation from the body and the body's preferences. Play-Doh, air dry clay, model magic, and other clay options can be positive ways to introduce texture and movement. Ripping and manipulating tissue paper or newspaper also give different sensations and can be utilized later in art pieces to repurpose and to refocus these movements. At this stage, I don't tend to bring in more fluid materials such as watercolor or other paint due to the difficulty with control. These introductions are quite slow and gradual.

DOI: 10.4324/9781032695228-9

Music choice while making art is an option; I ask the client to bring musical selections into session as opposed to something I provide. Music can grate on someone's nerves incredibly quickly or operate a recall of a memory that may be negative. I ask that clients "play DJ." I know for myself and for clients in recovery that it can be damaging for a song associated with using behaviors to be brought into the therapeutic space. It can also be helpful after the therapeutic milieu becomes a safe container to potentially process the song and the memory, but this may not be ideal early in the therapeutic relationship. Music is an incredibly powerful way of offering regulation or stimulation that can be beautiful, especially in tandem with movement and artmaking in session.

Movement is something that I will also recommend or offer in small doses; I will offer a movement and then make sure that I am joining with the client to reduce embarrassment if there is self-consciousness around the body present. Alternatively, I may stand side by side or in front of a client with my back to them to alleviate a sensation of scrutiny and to increase feelings of partnership or to decrease perfectionism. Introductory movements might simply be progressive muscle relaxation, shoulder rolls, abbreviated sun salutations, seated cat/cow, or "legs up the wall" if a client is willing and clothing permits. In addition, child's pose between active and resting can provide a good awareness of what these small movements might shift; active entails sweeping the arms overhead and reaching away from the body while resting is bringing the arms alongside the body while in this kneeling position with the forehead gently touching the ground. I want to provide "warm-ups" with movement when moving into this area of the ETC.

To introduce the kinesthetic/ sensory level of the ETC through art materials with clients, utilizing the Scribble drawing can be helpful. The examples that I am discussing were completed by children and adolescents who had experienced numerous placements, physical and emotional abuse, neglect, medical trauma, bullying, etc.; they were in a residential setting while creating the scribbles and had uncertainty around permanency.

When working with scribbles, I often tape large-scale paper on a wall (easily cleanable is ideal). Incorporating movement at the onset is a beneficial practice prior to the artmaking. In these cases, we utilized "airplane arms" and "wet noodle arms" to warm up. Then we playfully explored the different smells of the scented markers, deciding if they were gross or if they were appealing. Not surprisingly, the black licorice marker was generally not a favorite. I asked each of the individuals to start with a dark-colored marker so that we could clearly see the lines; then I requested that they make scribbles on the paper until they felt like their body was ready to stop.

The first individual was tentative and hesitant to get started. They were concerned that they would mess up and were rocking back and forth on their feet. I mirrored their movements and we used the rocking back and forth for regulation. We took deep breaths, and then the client and I worked on a scribble drawing; the directive was just to "make loops and scribbles until you feel ready to stop." The client and I took a step back after the loops and lines created the foundation and then looked for images in the scribble. The client identified a bigmouthed fish that came forward in the imagery. Though this did not immediately connect to a narrative, it provided an excellent warm-up and offered a chance for laughter and greater regulation in the body. As the client stood back to survey the work, the client's repetitive movements had visibly slowed and their breathing was regular and even. The process was important; the product was not as much.

I worked with a younger child who we described as "pumping the gas and the brakes at the same time." This child presented with "an overactive motor," constantly zooming around the halls; one time they ran from the art therapy room down the stairs and out the emergency exit when they saw someone they recognized through the window down in the parking lot. Impulsivity and hypervigilance were paired with dissociation and disconnection with the body. During this session, the child shared the crystals they were growing, a gift from the on-site teacher. The client asked me to feel them; when I did, I was surprised because they were gummy. I made a face; the client was happy that I was "grossed out" and tried to put them on my arm. They then discussed how they had "AWOL'ed," running from the residential facility. They reportedly heard "five gunshots" and was scared enough that they said, "I will never AWOL again." We talked about other ways to try to cope with feeling sad, angry, disappointed, or fearful rather than running away. We tried the yoga "legs up the wall" pose; the client could not balance and then giggled too hard to balance. I laughed as we both tumbled over; it seemed we were both warmed up, and I suggested a scribble drawing. I gave the client a black marker and asked them to scribble on the paper without lifting the marker until the paper was full. I then asked if any shapes or designs were observable. They asked for a scented green marker because he remembered the mint smell from a previous session. They colored on the paper with a lot of energy, eventually scribbling and jumping up and down. They then asked for red to outline the edges.

The client drew on the door by accident and turned around with an "uh-oh," looking for my reaction. I had given a boundary of keeping the marker on the paper and gave a gentle reminder. They then did it again and wiped the mark with a finger, saying, "See, it comes right off." Then they began purposely creating more marks on the door; I sensed the "testing" that was happening. The client then asked for a yellow marker and said, "See, this one doesn't even show up on the door," and continued to color on the paper and some on the door. After there was no more space to color, the client turned around. I asked them how they were feeling; the client appeared tired suddenly and surprised by their tiredness. Almost every bit of the paper had been filled in. The client sat on the floor and appeared exhausted. Since the client was so often in a hypervigilant as well as dissociative state, not only unaware of body sensations and responses but also in overdrive, constantly scanning for danger, for them to have some connection with the body and then get a sense of exhaustion was useful. This client rarely slept or slept with one eye open, and a feeling of relief and an ability to let go of some of the anxious energy appeared productive.

The third scribble process was with an adolescent who rarely made eye contact given that their eyes were covered over by a heavy curtain of bangs. During this session, the client began by performing several magic tricks. These card tricks were difficult to accomplish and required coordination. We then did arm stretches to prepare for a scribble drawing. I chose this prompt because the client had voiced to the primary residential therapist the day prior that they feared doing art with her, because they felt that it moved too quickly. I knew that a scribble could remove some of this trepidation because it reduced performance anxiety and the fear of revealing too much. Unlike some scribble drawings I had witnessed, this client was meticulous in the creation of the image, never lifting the marker (following directions) and covering all areas of the page with a mazelike design. I was astonished; this was an extremely well-organized scribble. There was a controlled, rhythmic completion of the scribble. During this session, we did not have to talk but could instead work on expression on a metaverbal level; the client seemed relieved that there had been no pressure placed to process but just could experience an art intervention in a safe, noninvasive way. There were a few shy grins, and the client seemed pleased that they had been able to cover the majority of the page.

With these three examples, the individuals warmed up their bodies, engaged the sense of smell with the scented markers, and created art with no expectation. Understanding that somatic responses and processes carry as much value and weight as cognitive processes, I know that work was being done, though not one of the individuals gave me an account of trauma history or expressed emotions verbally. What I have come to understand is that there can be a subtle (or not subtle) somatic shift where repair may be happening that is not verbalized. The push for the story can be unsettling and retraumatizing; this is not to say that the story isn't important. It is just that there is a time and place for this that may be later in your trajectory with the client or perhaps years after you encounter the client. I cannot say enough about laying the groundwork by beginning to reacquaint a client with their bodies and with their senses. We avoid our bodies when they have held so much pain. Being in the body may be one of the scariest things that a person can experience, but eventually this is a rewarding rejoining. Scribbles can be useful with all ages and all abilities, making adaptations as needed; sometimes a story comes from the images that are seen in the scribble. Other times it might just be that a client feels more relaxed or reconnected with themselves and their imagination.

Scribbles are by no means the only way to move into the kinesthetic/sensory level and into sensory integration/regulatory processes. They are just a great and easy start. A client came into my office this week and decided they needed plaster strips and a mask form; they had been thinking about this at school and then just had the idea that this felt like the next step in art therapy. They worked with the plaster bandages, talking minimally and focusing intently on dipping the strips into the water, wringing out the excess, placing the strips onto the mask form, and then smoothing the strips with their fingers. This was methodical and rhythmic; when the layer was complete, the client wanted air dry clay to then put thin layers onto the bandages, smoothing the clay out and taking great care with creating the texture that they wanted to achieve. They had come into the session somewhat downcast and tired; they left smiling and excited. This doesn't always happen, but in this instance, there was positive benefit with the manipulation of the materials. The client's body knew what to ask for in the art therapy room.

Activating the kinesthetic/sensory and offering sensory integration through Play-Doh and model magic or additional 3D materials can be helpful. I had one client who spent 45 minutes working feverishly with Play-Doh and a plastic extruder kit, pushing and pulling the material until they had utilized all six containers of Play-Doh. They did not pause or look up during the process until all of the materials were utilized; at that point, they looked at me, thanked me, and left the room. With another client, they utilized watercolor and practiced with letting the watercolor drip and flow on the paper. The watched as the watercolors made rivulets on the page but then decided upon creating a large tree in the center. This was a large sheet of paper which allowed for greater movements with the arms and fluidity with the medium. The client created a large redwood tree with a lake near it, voicing that like the redwood, he felt strong and that with water nearby, he was not worried about fires. Since he was returning home soon from his placement, he was able to talk about how fear had often led to anger at home. We were able to write a plan out about communicating fear and anger in ways that others might be able to better understand; we shared this with the community in which the client lived to help ease the client's transition.

It is also in this phase of the ETC where often parents, colleagues, teachers, clients, and caregivers ask the question, "What exactly is happening in session?" Looking at scribbles or piles of Play-Doh, scented markers, or sensory materials, there isn't a "product" necessarily. It can appear that play is happening or simple experimentation, which can be perceived as non-useful or not productive by individuals unfamiliar with trauma work and art therapy. Being able to explain the value of repair utilizing play and art interventions to family members and to treatment teams is essential in order to increase buy in to the therapeutic process as well as to encourage play and to provide an invitation for play and art in other settings. I remember having a client who asked to go outside and throw model magic at a tree and yell; another client was making an art piece by dipping their hands in paint, experimenting with the sensation of the paint on their hands, and then making handprints on a huge piece of cardboard in the parking lot of the group practice where I was working. There were a few blue handprints on doorknobs that required some cleanup afterward! Sometimes caregivers, relationship partners, and even colleagues want quick fixes or quick explanations for what is happening in session.

There is work happening here, important work. The body is coming back online through rhythms, sensory exploration and curiosity, and movements that are awakening the breath. When trauma occurs, we work very hard to separate from our bodies to cease the pain from happening. It can be difficult to explain that a seed is being planted to pave the road for deepening and trauma repair. This is a stage setting, but it is as equally important as the phases to follow; there is repair happening in the experimentation, the movement, the engaging of curiosity, and hopefully a reconnection to play and openness to newness. "Art activities that involve repetition and positive sensory sensations soothe the lower parts of the brain, reduce stress responses, enhance self-regulation, and slow down the sympathetic nervous system; they also nonverbally communicate that life is stable and consistent" (Malchiodi, 2014, pp. 58–59).

When individuals have questions about what is happening in session during this stage, I explain that we are activating the kinesthetic/sensory levels of the Expressive Therapies Continuum and engaging the first domain of the Neurosequential Model of Therapeutics. It is helpful to have a neuroscience-based response to have on the ready. Remembering that cumulative trauma repair occurs on a continuum, it may be challenging to discern the level or the domain as they often happen concurrently. In the examples given, the sensory integration areas have been emphasized. Often sensory integration and kinesthetic/sensory levels quickly open the pathway for regulation and potentially meaning making, which is a higher-level executive function.

References

Elbrecht, C. (2018). *Healing trauma with guided drawing: A Sensorimotor art therapy approach to bilateral body mapping.* Berkeley, CA: North Atlantic Books.

Malchiodi, C. A. (2014). *Creative arts and play therapy for attachment problems.* New York: The Guilford Press.

7 Engaging Emotional Regulation and Perceptual/ Affective Levels of the Expressive Therapies Continuum

When we move into the process of emotional regulation and eventually self-regulation and self-soothing, the client begins to potentially experience a bit of relief and regains episodes of greater control over somatic responses and emotional expression. Malchiodi states that supporting "an internal sense of stabilization" through an introduction of therapeutic interventions that assist with self-regulation is essential prior to exploring the traumatic events themselves (2020, p. 165). It can be argued as well that the repair may or may not be in the storytelling but more in the repair of somatic experiences, not to discount the importance of the story or the release of a series of narratives.

This is where the movements and art explorations begin to have an impact on the body and the breath, and both the client and the therapist can reflect on co-regulatory processes engaged in session. Utilizing the examples of the scribbles previously, the "fish scribble" went from sensorimotor activity, rocking, exploration of color, and scents to then looking at mark making to color in loops and to find shapes. The second scribble that began as a product of motor agitation and explosion on the page eventually slowed down to coloring more intentionally with greater choice around color options and more intentional filling in of spaces. The client became more relaxed, appearing almost fatigued after the expulsion of energy and the bringing of the body to a more regulated state. The last scribble was intentional to begin with, and the client remained regulated as they worked throughout the process.

With the snake example, the client was able to progress from the simple rolling of the clay back and forth to creating a shape, adding stripes of a different color of clay to the form, and adding dots/eyes with marker. The client with the Play-Doh and the extruder began to slow frenzied movements and energy exertion to a more rhythmic and regulated state. The caregiver mentioned that they took a nap as soon as the session was complete.

It is at this point in the process when working with breathing skills and identifying areas of regulation (looseness) in the body versus areas that feel activated (constricted, tense, overly active, hot, etc.) are useful. I consider this an opportunity to try to "grow" the areas of regulation into the areas that feel

DOI: 10.4324/9781032695228-10

dysregulated. There are many approaches to this, but I will offer just a few that I have accumulated along the way. One thing that can be daunting is asking clients to move into somatic work by immediately introducing body scans or small body maps. I generally will start with external imaging first to grow comfortability; in telehealth or as a homework assignment, I have asked clients to go on a scavenger hunt in their homes or outside to look for objects that have a positive connection and then another object that has either a neutral or a slightly less positive connection. It is important that the client be aware that this is not to go to something that is connected to a traumatic or triggering experience. We then will play with physical and somatic sensations in relation to the objects and then utilize the resource object (positive) to help with addressing the less positive option. Asking the client to just experience these options and to notice sensations and then lean into a positive resource to help with regulation can bring awareness to areas of the body that can be helpful with greater self-regulation. Oscillation or pendulation between these options can bring a sense of homeostasis and an improved ability to self soothe.

If clients are able to go into the body a little bit, I offer circles, small body maps, boxes, an old book for altered book projects, etc., to offer a sense of containment and to begin with a creation of transitional objects for resources inside and outside of the session. To start, drawing a circle on a piece of paper is a bit of magic that I find intriguing. Many of you have probably seen the videos of a circle drawn around an ant where the ant then wanders around the inside of the circle but does not move outside of the edges of the shape. If you compare getting a blank piece of paper to begin with versus one with a circle drawn on it, it can elicit starkly different responses. The circle gives an imaginal container for a client to fill in without dealing with simply blank space. Asking a client to fill the circle in with colors, shapes, and lines gives an entry way into the perceptive/affective levels. I wonder if the heart and brain wander around the inside of the circle much like the ant; this intervention allows for somatic and emotional expression with a boundary to hold the expressions of emotion and to offer a symbolic regulatory process. If clients want to expand and draw around the outside or manipulate the paper and become more curious/experimental, I welcome that in the session.

Alternatively, the third picture directive for the Diagnostic Drawing Series (DDS) is "The Feeling Picture," and the directive is to "Make a picture of how you're feeling, using lines, shapes, and colors." A semi-structured task, it asks the client to communicate about their affective state directly, as well as to represent it in abstract form (Cohen & Mills, 2016). Individuals are directed to draw on 18″ × 24″ inch paper with chalk pastels (12 color pack). For individuals who are well versed in art materials or have few reservations about utilizing large paper with messier materials, this can be amazing to explore the perceptual/affective level. However, having taught Assessment and Appraisal in Art Therapy, I found that even graduate-level art therapy students at times were tentative with this part of the DDS, finding it to be "too abstract" or drawing in only one small corner of the paper. For individuals who have experienced trauma, moving into chalk pastels, large paper, and abstract concepts around emotion can be challenging.

This is where I provide materials that may give the ability to work in the abstract but do so with more structure, foundation, and containment. I utilize shoe boxes, smaller jewelry-sized boxes, origami boxes, etc., during sessions to work with regulatory practice. Simply painting or embellishing containers with paint, stickers, collage materials, etc., offers choice, repetitive movement, and containment. Bringing attention to how it feels to work on the outside of the container versus the inside can also bring awareness to external/internal somatic responses. Containers present a client with an increased sense of structure and containment when hypervigilance/dissociation has previously been the default mode. They can also experience themselves on the inside or the outside of the container with less risk.

Tissue paper or multicolored paper collage allows for choice of color and texture. I love asking a client to match colors of tissue paper to their feelings and then create a collage utilizing those colors of tissue paper. I will ask clients if they are able to consider how often and how strongly they may experience the emotions and then to consider that in their imagery, creating an emotional map of sorts. By being able to manipulate the tissue paper by tearing, gluing, smashing, wadding up/pulling back open, folding, etc., this allows for regulatory opportunities and abstract representation of emotional states.

I do utilize small body maps when I have enough familiarity with a client to predict the efficacy and the safety of this intervention. Rarely do I practice large body tracing as this requires a physical proximity and a potentially distorted representation of a client, which could trigger either negative body image or traumatic recall. With body maps, I typically offer a gingerbread person outline or an ambiguous figure outline; with these, I invite an individual to create colors and shapes to indicate areas of the body that feel positive or relaxed, considering temperature/texture etc. Then if the client presents as regulated, I will invite them to indicate areas that may feel less pleasant (blocked, restricted, painful, etc.). This can be done on the same image or giving the client two outlines (one for the resource areas of the body and one for the less pleasant). If this is done on two, then the client can turn the negative one over and spend time with the positive and vice versa. This allows for control, oscillation between sensations, and resourcing. This is where asking the client to change their physical sensations by utilizing imagery and mark making gives the client a sense of greater self-regulation. I will typically mirror movements and work to regulate my system to offer co-regulation throughout the process.

Offering walking, simple yoga poses (asanas), sand tray, and sensory items is also integral for regulation though perhaps less so in conjunction with the perceptual/affective levels of the Expressive Therapies Continuum (ETC) except for introducing more comfortability with the body, enhancing capacity for artmaking. In the previous chapter, I discussed airplane arms, noodle arms, etc. Kathy Higby, a colleague and dear friend, asks clients to "walk their feet" and to "let the body breathe you." I have shared multiple times the walking of the feet as it is incredibly helpful as a tool that can be done anywhere from a difficult work meeting or a challenging social encounter. This is a simple alternation between a heel toe movement on the left foot to the right foot that causes a calming sensation for the body and a reminder for the breath to become more even. The book, *Breathe like a Bear*, has excellent recommendations for simple breathing regulatory practices that are accessible for all ages with lovely illustrations.

We may use legs up the wall, sun salutations, and child's pose quite frequently, but I am also careful not to move people into movement too quickly as some yoga positions can leave a client feeling vulnerable. Ellen Horovitz's *Head and Heart: Yoga Therapy and Art Therapy Interventions for Mental Health* is a beautiful resource for these types of interventions. As I mentioned before, utilizing child's pose as an example, sweeping the arms above the head for the active version of the pose and then sweeping the arms back toward the hips is the passive form; asking a client to pendulate between the two and just note the sensations in the body awakens the ability to discern small distinctions.

In my office, I also have bins of different types of balls and squeezy toys as well as rocks and natural elements. Just experiencing different textures, weights, temperatures, and then shifting between these elements can offer regulatory processes. I have spent numerous sessions with individuals sitting on the floor rolling a ball back and forth between us and practicing breathing; I have sensed an increase in rapport and regulation, trust-building, and alliance creation. Going through your life with the understanding that there isn't anyone who would reciprocate your feelings or bother to respond to you can stunt socioemotional development; it make take some time before there is a sense that the person on the other side of the ball might be trustworthy enough to play with or that they won't cause you harm in some way. After all, I believe most of us want reciprocity and emotional intimacy in relationships, but that capacity may not have been cultivated or supported. Through a greater sense of sensory integration, emotional regulation, and access to the kinesthetic/ sensory, perceptual/affective levels, an evolution toward alliance building and greater relational capacity can be bridged.

References

Cohen, B. M., & Mills, A. (2016). The Diagnostic Drawing Series (DDS) at thirty: Art therapy assessment and research. In D. E. Gussak & M. L. Rosal (Eds.), *The Wiley handbook of art therapy* (pp. 558–568). Malden, MA: Wiley Blackwell.

Malchiodi, C. A. (2020). *Trauma and expressive arts therapy: Brain, body, and imagination in the healing process: Brain, body, and imagination in the healing process.* New York: The Guilford Press.

Part IV
Building the Therapeutic Alliance and Relational Capacity

8 Art Media and Art Interventions That Will Enhance the Therapeutic Alliance

As we move toward the cognitive/symbolic levels of the Expressive Therapies Continuum (ETC) and the cognitive/executive functioning areas of Neuro-sequential Model of Therapeutics (NMT), it feels important to discuss the building of the therapeutic alliance and relational capacity. Engaging regulatory practices first that increase sensory awareness and integration will assist in relational capacity building. What does rapport-building look like with art media in session? In this chapter, examining how to join in relationally and to create greater equality through collaborative engagement will be explored. In addition, there will be a discussion of group therapy versus individual therapy practices; when is it appropriate for individuals to move into group therapy? When we consider the word "resistant" as practitioners, what do we really mean? To increase engagement and the beneficial qualities of a therapeutic alliance, moving out of a power differential and into a collaborative approach is essential; this means meeting a client in correlation to and with developmental level, which can be impacted by the effects of cumulative trauma.

Due to financial constraints, evidence-based treatment models, accessibility, and a shortage of therapists, very often individuals are brought into the treatment setting and immediately placed into groups. I have seen this in substance abuse, eating disorder, problem sexual behavior, and even trauma treatment settings where clients are placed in groups before ever having access to individual settings. Though this may be appropriate and useful for many clients, those with relational and cumulative trauma may not receive benefit from the group setting initially and could potentially sustain further harm. Dayton writes in her relational trauma training manual that we act out our family dynamics, ruptures, etc., within present-day relational systems. Since we don't have a context for what happens in our childhood and adolescent memories due to the need to disconnect from our bodies, the memories live in the body in a disorganized fashion, in "wordless sense impressions." We avoid groups of people, perhaps people in general, since they are the source of pain and of rupture. Reintroduction to relationship in safe ways needs to happen slowly and gradually. Given that the pain and the intergenerational trauma occur relationally, the healing needs to take place relationally (Dayton, 2023).

DOI: 10.4324/9781032695228-12

While I was teaching a supervision course to art therapy graduate students, we began discussing what makes supervision feel productive and equitable; how does the container feel safe enough to delve into areas of transference and countertransference as well as exploring potential "imposter syndrome" or perfectionism showing up in the early stages of their careers? One of the students mentioned that they appreciated that I "joined in" by creating artwork alongside them and that I was willing to share and to discuss my work and to receive feedback from my students. We discussed the importance of belonging and of being seen through compassionate and loving eyes. If this is important for developing art therapists, it feels equally essential in laying the groundwork within the therapeutic alliance.

The Physical Container

Hermanson (2009) offers guidelines around creating a container; this is in the context of teaching and mentoring, but it feels applicable to the therapeutic milieu. She begins with the physical; what does the space look like and feel like? Is it inviting and can the client see themselves in or connect with something in the space? This is as important through Zoom as it is in the physical space; what does your background say about you and how you welcome someone in? I remember at the beginning of the pandemic having a meeting with a colleague who had a background with a gorgeous, white, glowing apartment with an incredible view, not realizing that this was a background filter. I spent the meeting wondering how they kept the space looking so clean, so perfect, and so expensive rather than focusing on the topic at hand. The perfection of the background was distracting and distancing for me.

There won't be a physical container that is welcoming to everyone, but I do think having elements of self and elements of safety in the space can be useful. I have an "office tortoise" named Prince who greets everyone by the door in his crate; he has artwork that has been created by various clients posted all over and around the crate in his honor. The comments are generally that the office feels like a home rather than an office. I acknowledge that having a safe and comfortable place to practice is a privilege and that, by offering this space with the hope of it being welcoming, I am aware that it is through socioeconomic and educational privilege that I can do so. For art therapists, we require supplies to be able to offer choice and to effectively integrate all aspects of the ETC. This can be expensive; at the onset of my career, I remember many sites wanting an art therapist but not understanding that art supplies were needed. This meant having fundraising events, emailing all staff begging for recyclables or unwanted materials, dollar store runs, garage sales, etc.

While working in different agencies, there wasn't always freedom to create the ideal physical space. I remember working in a closet-sized office with no windows; I created a painting of a window to put on the wall, but that was a tough space to enhance. There were instances due to safety concerns in residential settings where there were limitations to space, and just finding an empty area to have a session with some semblance of confidentiality was a challenge. Doing home counseling meant that sessions were often held in kitchens, living rooms, doctor's office waiting areas, cars, libraries, and fast-food parking lots. Sometimes the container is the therapeutic alliance versus the physical space. The ability to regulate your physical and somatic self in environments that may or may not be conducive to alliance-building is a skill. Though the physical space is important, the intersubjective space between the client and the therapist and additionally the artwork is integral, no matter the environment.

The physical container can become more challenging while doing family or group therapy. It can be difficult to offer a configuration that enhances the container for a family system or group members that also accommodates art-making. In my office, I have a large table that will fit six to seven individuals and still allow for personal space/space for creation. However, in previous situations, this could look like group members working in areas on the floor, areas outside, group projects that were taped to the wall, and then a lot of moving of furniture and returning to a circle to process the artmaking as a whole.

The Conceptual and Ideological Container

Skaife (2001) wrote:

What is made in art therapy derives its meaning from the intersubjective space within which it is made, and this space unfolds within time. Within this time frame, the gesture made, for example, the brushstroke or the impression of the hand within the clay, is the language, the expression, rather than it being the translation of an idea of a thought. The making of the artwork, its facture, is its meaning. We only find what we want to say in saying it. In making art we never arrive at a representation of an inner image; the inner image is shaped by what it is we make and is entirely dependent on it. We only understand the artwork through our active engagement with it, its meaning is in what it does to the intersubjective space in which it is seen. The origin of the work of art does not solely reside within the artist.

(p. 46)

In art therapy, the understanding of intersubjective space between the creator and the art piece, the therapist and the client, and the therapist and the art piece offers multiple connections and an ideological framework for the therapeutic container. Hermanson (2009) discusses conceptual and ideological containers for teaching; when applied to the therapeutic alliance, having the framework for therapy that is transparent and collaborative in nature inspires a greater sense of trust, purpose, and direction. Depending on the setting, the biopsychosocial assessment process is generally the first component of the therapeutic process. For many clinicians including myself, this needs to be completed within the first session and involves a provisional diagnosis. We work collaboratively on the kindest, gentlest, and most accurate diagnosis, knowing that this is a fluid process that could shift as we get to know each other. I want to build rapport during the biopsychosocial assessment process but offering a sense of humor, operating from a strength-based perspective, and utilizing unconditional, positive regard.

The diagnosis (if applicable) and the treatment plan are the foundational elements that provide structure and scaffolding for the journey together. I have experienced too many clients coming into the therapeutic space who take psychotropic medications with no idea of diagnosis or even what the medication is designed to address. In the context of cumulative trauma, clients tend to enter a process with me after multiple treatment avenues, levels of care, and medications without an idea of what they were doing, the direction they were going, or a greater understanding of self. Cumulative trauma symptoms and behaviors can present as or be comorbid with many other diagnoses or survival skills that can be difficult to discern. I know with my own treatment progression, I was misdiagnosed on numerous occasions until I found a provider who felt more aligned with trauma repair and well versed in the constellation of trauma symptomology.

I may or may not utilize art therapy directives to construct the treatment plan depending on the client's preferences and comfortability with the art process; however, there are a few directives that I feel lay the groundwork to begin the process efficiently and creatively. One is a modified road drawing process based on Hanes's road drawing assessment (1997). I will offer a medium-sized sheet of white paper and oil pastels, markers, colored pencils, crayons, etc., and ask the individual to work in stages:

1   Draw a road on the page.
2   Create an environment around the road.
3   Draw yourself somewhere in the picture.
4   Draw three barriers that could get in the way on the journey.
5   Draw three resources (people, places, things, animals, etc.) that could be helpful on the journey.

When we process the image, we discuss how the road feels, whether the client is on the road, and how their symbol is supported (or not supported) in the environment. How does the environment feel? Did they draw themselves or a symbol for themselves? Are the barriers relatable to something in their present-day reality/world? Do the resources exist in the present-day world, or do the resources need to be bolstered? This conversation generally leads nicely into creating three treatment goals and three objectives. When utilizing this directive in a family process or in a group setting, it can be incredible to watch group members offer suggestions, make observations, and create individual goals as well as collective goals.

I had an adolescent client who drew a windy road that went from one corner to the opposite corner; the figure they drew was not on the road but in the woods, building a fire. There were potholes, caution tape, and police all along the road. The figure surrounded by trees had a backpack. When asked about the backpack, the client stated that they "cheated" by having multiple resources in the bag (cell phone with friends' contact info, water, unlimited food, books, music, plushies, etc.). We talked about being well prepared rather than cheating and talked about how smart this figure was to find their own space away from the barriers. We also discovered that the barriers were not of their own making, and these were things the client was needing to avoid, to escape in her own environment. They were having nightmares and losing sleep, experiencing flashbacks and hypervigilance and, at times, dissociating. We discussed the survival skills that had once been helpful but had started to lose the usefulness and were becoming detrimental. From this, we created treatment goals that amplified existing strengths and decreased trauma responses by identifying triggering factors and coming up with coping options.

Emotional landscape drawings, paintings, collages, etc., are also helpful for treatment planning and identifying the treatment trajectory. For the emotional landscape, the directive is to draw, paint, collage, etc., your emotions as if they were a landscape image. I try to put this into more concrete language and elaborate by asking questions such as, what type of weather would your feelings be? Would there be lakes or desert, mountains or flat surfaces? This can be helpful to literally get an idea of the terrain. One little boy drew tornados all over his image; he stated that everyone in his house was angry and that he was angry too. This led to a conversation of what the tornadoes might need to express their anger in less destructive ways as well as what other emotions could be present for the tornadoes. We worked on treatment goals for the family and for the client based on this image. The emotional landscape drawing was an excellent starting point with a group of 15–20 boys, 11–14 years old, in an after-school group that I conducted annually for a number of years. We pinned all the completed images on the board and talked about how it would feel if all of the weather patterns and landscapes existed in the same scene. The boys talked about how it would probably be "crazy" and overwhelming considering the number of volcanoes and storms in the pictures. We discussed what we would all need to be in the same landscape together to feel safe and to feel like we could talk openly. This led to creating group goals and guidelines and a conceptual framework.

Lastly, my favorite way of working on treatment planning comes from simply drawing a series of emotions. This can be done with two, four, six, or eight images depending on time, attention span, and need. I offer either separate sheets of paper (usually small squares 4″× 4″ or 6″× 6″) or one large sheet of paper folded into up to eight squarish rectangles and unfolded to reveal the crease lines. I offer choice around material between watercolor, oil pastels, colored pencils, markers, and crayons. This could also be done three-dimensionally with clay or model magic. I then ask the individual to start by drawing happy if it jumped out of their body and landed on the page. I do stipulate not using faces or words to allow for more creativity and less reliance on emojis and stereotypical imagery. If a client is struggling with the abstract nature of this, I will alter the directive slightly by suggesting an image of something that gives them the feeling of happy. From the feeling of happy, I generally alternate between what is conceived to be pleasurable emotions and then perhaps less enjoyable feelings. We move to sad, then excited, then angry, peaceful, scared, etc. I will usually leave the last space for a feeling the client experiences but that I didn't mention prior. Also, if the client has voiced anxiety or depression, I will substitute depressed for sad, anxious for scared. For many clients, happy might be a very difficult feeling to get reacquainted with; sometimes sad, angry, anxious, scared, etc., can be more accessible and easier to represent. This may take one to possibly three sessions depending on the depth of the processing and the speed of the creator. If this feels possible, we discuss somatic associations and experiences with the emotions as they are created. Oscillating between the emotional states can be useful for resourcing and for regulation. Through pendulating between the feelings states, it can then be possible to think about "growing" joyful emotions and either decreasing painful feelings or expressing them in healthy ways. Through this process treatment goals can be established in individualized and creative pathways.

Additionally, this can be effective in family and group settings. I prefer using the small squares to process slightly differently. I will ask the members to put their initials on the backs of each square before starting; we then move through the feelings and talk about the imagery as a collective. We will put all the happy squares together, sad squares, etc., and then discuss similarities and differences between form, lines, and color for each emotional state. This helps with cultivating cohesion and to recognize that we all have the feelings and that these feelings could be similar or different in the way we experience them together or separately. It is a good springboard for discussing what people may need when they are in these emotional states and how others could respond in helpful and meaningful ways.

Revisiting Sensory Integration and Emotional Regulation

At this point, you may be wondering, what happened to this sensory integration and emotional regulation prep work discussed in prior chapters? Yes, this is the conundrum of practice and what is clinically indicated versus what is dictated by managed care. In a perfect world, there would be multiple opportunities for sensory integration, emotional regulation, and relational capacity building in a lovely, linear, orderly fashion; what I find is that in most therapeutic settings, we have to adapt and layer the four functional domains often all within the first couple of sessions. By offering the treatment planning process through creative avenues that engage the ETC, my hope is that we can build in sensory enriched and regulatory options while completing the treatment plan. Since creating a treatment plan in a collaborative way requires a partnership as well as cognitive functioning, it is important to provide opportunities for regulation and integration along the way. I find that after completing the biopsychosocial and the treatment plan, we can step back further into the sensory integration and emotional regulation domains with the "bones" in place to provide direction for our time together.

References

Dayton, T. (2023). *Relational trauma treatment workshop processing deep childhood wounds with psychodrama and experiential relational trauma: Psychodrama and experiential interventions for treating childhood wounds in adult clients.* Eau Claire, WI: PESI, Inc.

Hanes, M. (1997). *Roads to the unconscious: A manual for understanding road drawings.* Oklahoma City: Wood N. Barnes.

Hermanson, K. (2009). *Getting messy: A Guide to taking risks and opening the imagination for teachers, trainers, coaches, and mentors.* San Rafael, CA: Rawberry Books.

Skaife, S. (2001). Making visible: Art therapy and intersubjectivity. *Inscape, 6*(2), 40–50. https://doi.org/10.1080/17454830108414030

9 The Artwork as Container

Defining Safety and Creating Safety

Creating opportunities for container building and for explorations of safety on micro and macro levels is one of my favorite aspects of the therapeutic process. I treasure these processes, because they can be longer range, ongoing alliance-building journeys. They can become transitional objects from "outside life" to the therapeutic milieu; clients tend to look forward to coming in to be able to work on their art and reflect upon how they thought about what they wanted to do next or what they had done the previous week throughout their time in between sessions. If these are processes that are worked on at home, it provides a window into the events, feelings, and emotional states between therapist and client meetings.

> In the dynamic equilibrium between a relatively fluid self and reality, transitional objects are not limited to childhood but continue into adolescence and adulthood. Transitional objects chosen by an individual may represent that individual and aid in feelings of self-continuity and control.
>
> (McCullough, 2009)

The importance of feeling "in control" provides a greater sense of safety and self-concept no matter the external setting. Safety is a deeply personal and individuated experience; there is no clear definition or art practice/art experience that will offer this for every person. However, providing containers and options for collaboration can be useful. It is essential to consider cultural, family of origin, and trauma backgrounds when offering options. I will discuss a few options that I will tend to offer, though there is a much wider array in art therapy practice available.

Altered Books

Jacobson-Levy and Miller (2022) describe the process of altered book making as activating destruction in a contained fashion within the book and its pages.

> As the book's content and structure are dismantled, the artist's personal narrative emerges and transforms the original book. This metamorphosis is

DOI: 10.4324/9781032695228-13

inherent in the creation of an altered book. The act of rebuilding involves making internal or external repairs and restorations to a circumstance, structure, or form that has been damaged, broken, or impaired. In therapy, rebuilding may look like mending fractured relationships with the self and others, finding a sense of emotional resolve, recovery in the wake of adversity, or managing a major life change.

(p. 195)

Themes of creative destruction, reforming, reclaiming, and transformation can be explored.

When offering this process, I either request that the client finds a book for themselves (from something they are willing to reimagine or a book that they purchase or find used) or I provide a number of choices being careful to have a wide selection of possibilities. One thing to note is that the destruction and reconstruction of a book may not be acceptable or respectful depending on culture, possible scarcity of books, and reverence for the written word. Checking this out with the client beforehand is important. I want the client to feel in control and to feel confident about moving into the process; for some individuals, it may feel freeing to be able to destroy to create, while for others, this could be daunting or subversive in some way.

When moving forward, I offer several materials such as collage, paint, colored pencil, markers, Posca paint pens, etc., so that the client can decide where they would like to be with the Expressive Therapies Continuum (more fluid, less fluid, more controlled, less controlled). This will most likely shift from session to session or if the client is working at home after initiating the process in session. The choice of next steps after the book and the materials is initially selected for the beginning of the process and then makes way into theme selection. Clients may want to work without a theme or prompts or may seek or desire direction. What is most important is the option to rewrite a narrative, whether this stems from the narrative that exists in the book itself that becomes connected to the client's own metaphorical narrative or if this is imposed on the book from the client to more directly recreate and to transform their own personal story. With cumulative trauma, the ability to utilize a "magic wand" to rewrite on a somatic and symbolic level their own past, present, and future can present an opportunity for repair and for transformation. Most importantly, the client can close the book or open the book, destroy, or create/recreate. They can choose the trajectory of the story and the process, having ultimate autonomy with their book and their narrative. This can be restorative by trading lack of control for absolute control, even if this merely metaphorical is embodied.

Circle Drawings and Circle Journals

During my first two years of being an art therapist and a counselor, I was finding that I was struggling with sleep and with regulation. I had nightmares about experiences that happened in the workplace or areas of countertransference stemming from parallels in clients' cumulative trauma experiences with my own. I had started a circle journal in graduate school and then restarted the process, noting that nightmares discontinued and that I was better able to put the experiences of the day behind me once the work hours were over. Each day, I would draw a circle on a page of the journal and then fill the circle with my thoughts, feelings, and somatic states; completing the image and then closing the journal helped me have a conclusion to the day. I have provided clients with journals or asked them to find one that fits them and do a similar process for themselves if it felt helpful. I noted that in my practice, this was particularly effective with reducing behaviors related to process addictions, substance use, self-harm, and disordered eating. There was a reduction in the need to self-medicate and the ability to self-regulate in a conscious and contained fashion.

In sessions, I utilize circle drawings with different directives depending on the need of the client. I remember I had one client who would come in and feel that the time we had together could not possibly hold all the moments of the previous week that felt important to disclose. She would recount the events in a pressured and rapid-fire way that did not allow time for reflection or reparative options. After several sessions of experiencing what seemed to be verbal regurgitation for both of us, I offered a circle, asking the client to write or draw words/symbols of everything that was in her head at that moment. Then I asked her to circle or star the top three priorities for the session; we then spent some time with those three areas with ample time for reflection and for emotional regulation. This then became the framework for our sessions; the client's response to this was far more positive. She also started to use this practice for problem-solving and for self-reflection independently.

I like to use circles for boundary work; what are the people, places, emotions, experiences, objects, etc., that the client would like in the circle with them versus the people, places, emotions, experiences, objects, etc., that they would prefer to have outside of the circle? How can the individual fortify these boundaries? Can we play around with how it feels to bring some things inside of the circle or trade them with things inside the circle? If the client doesn't want to draw, consider utilizing a Hula-Hoop; the client can stand in the Hula-Hoop and write on Post-its or index cards, moving the different elements inside or outside of the Hula-Hoop. Being able to "play" with boundaries and experience/embody them through metaphorical means can create a greater sense of control and of safety.

Containers

Utilizing different types of containers offers the ability to hold emotions, sensations, and memories that could otherwise feel overwhelming, potentially leading to hyper- or hypo-arousal. Containers offer the ability to engage with the possibly triggering pieces but with distance and without having to actively tell the story. For example, one option is to ask the individual to choose a rock (I have a bowl of differently shaped, textured, and hued rocks) and then ask the client to create a safe space for the rock. I offer recyclables, paper, tissue paper, wood pieces, etc., but this would also be good with an outdoor scavenger hunt to find elements in nature. This intervention offers the ability to create safety and to design what safety could look like even if the individual isn't entirely familiar with the sensation of safety. It allows for an individual to have some control over building safety and regulation; if the client is able and is regulated, we can move into discussing how it feels to be the rock in this space and what it might be like to have this space in reality/how to build this space. However, if the client is not able to "go there," there is still a felt sense or embodied sense of this concept.

Natural element jars can be useful and can give a link to the natural world that could be rejuvenating or soothing. You can go for a walk with your client or you can assign a walk for your client (environment and safety allowing), picking up random pieces that call to you and your client and then considering how these could be placed in a clear container or a box for the client to revisit when needed. Gavron and Shemesh (2022) discussed the merits of creating terrariums as a nature-based art therapy intervention to foster a multilayered exploration of a personal space and a symbolic visual story. Through this process, the participants in the study were able to create multidimensional miniature worlds to consider past, present, and future and to increase autonomy. If natural elements and terrariums are impossible given surroundings and circumstances, found object jars can be substituted and can work for telehealth. With these, I will ask a client to locate a container that will hold found elements in their environment and then consider how those elements work together in the container. If the objects elicit memories, this could offer a safer experience of processing the memories or exploring the symbolism. Most importantly, the creator of these containers has the ability to omit or to include what they desire. They can control the miniature world, and they have choice around every element. In a world where sometimes choice, collaboration, and control can feel elusive, this process allows for a greater sense of power. When processing, it is helpful to discuss where areas of power can be found "in the real world" and how feelings of security and self-advocacy can be developed or further increased.

References

Gavron, T., & Shemesh, H. (2022). "I am actually growing my art": Expressive terrarium as an intervention tool in arts therapy. *Journal of Creativity in Mental Health. 19*(1), 24–38. https://doi.org/10.1080/15401383.2022.2119184

Jacobson-Levy, M., & Miller, G. M. (2022). Creative destruction in art and therapy: Reframing, reforming, reclaiming. *Art Therapy: Journal of the American Art Therapy Association, 39*(4), 194–202. https://doi.org/10.1080/07421656.2022.2090306

McCullough, C. (2009). A child's use of transitional objects in art therapy to cope with divorce. *Art Therapy: Journal of the American Art Therapy Association, 26*(1), 19–25. https://doi.org/10.1080/07421656.2009.10129306

Part V

Embracing the Cognitive/Symbolic and the Creative Levels

Part V

Embracing the
Cognitive\Symbolic and
the Creative\Carols

10 Bridging the Bottom-Up and the Top-Down Through Oscillation and Metaphoric Meaning Making

While supervising students engaged in the fieldwork portion of graduate level education as well as supervisees seeking licensure, there is a desire to "get to the work," to the meaning making and the cognitive/symbolic level or the fluidity of the creative levels of the Expressive Therapies Continuum (ETC) and the Neurosequential Model of Therapeutics. The reminder to slow down, to attend to the bottom-up processes first is not only essential but also in no way linear. Looking at the ETC as an interconnected circle versus as a hierarchical system is helpful when considering cultural reflexivity and attending to the impact of one level upon another; balance is essential, and the lack of development or engagement in one area impacts the ability to engage in another.

> Expression and interaction on the different levels of the ETC involve information intrinsic and unique to each level; at the same time, the levels are interrelated causing successive changes. For example, the successful completion of a safe place drawing (a Symbolic activity) may elicit feelings of safety and calm.
>
> (Hinz, Rim, & Lusebrink, 2022, p. 3)

Conversely, if a person is dysregulated and attempting to create the symbol of a safe place, this may or may not be achieved and may not be embodied or somatically experienced.

Speaking to the culturally reflexive nature of the circular ETC model and to bridging the bottom-up and top-down processes, Taylor-Johnson (2023) recounted her own heuristic research experience regarding her knitting process:

> Knitting offered the opportunities to sit with the sense of being and emotional upheaval. The project allowed for the development of wellness and boundaries, I found myself better able to navigate daily microaggressions, and create a sense of safety. There were moments that allowed for me to check in with myself beyond the knitting. While making somatic art as

DOI: 10.4324/9781032695228-15

a response to these check-ins was profound, it was in the daily practice of becoming attuned that allowed me to set quicker boundaries with increased firmness.

(p. 18)

The author was able to connect the somatic process of knitting with direct application to her daily experience of living, recounting that this project aided with identity exploration, emotional reflection, mindfulness, and community integration. Ultimately, however, the process connected to storytelling and to the woven intersubjectivity of her own story with that of her father's and the overall stories of community. By connecting the levels of the ETC, there was the option to operate on all levels simultaneously, allowing for the space for creativity and artistic flow while also providing room for direct application in daily living and in relationship construction.

I find that giving the client/artist the opportunity to find their own way to the cognitive/symbolic and ultimately the creative space is most helpful. I can offer supplies and options that may cultivate the possibility for this movement, but I'm not driving the car so to speak. Sometimes when clients first come in, there is a misconception that art therapists are meant to interpret their artwork or to read their imagery like reading tea leaves or a psychic phenomenon of sorts. At times, I've noticed some disappointment when I stated that I would help them to recognize their own personal symbology in partnership with them versus inserting my own opinions about what their imagery means. In other instances, I've asked about the meaning of a portion of an image or asked about the function of a part of a drawing to be met with, "that's just a tree (or whatever the literal representation of the art is)." This feels like a small rupture but can be repaired easily with acceptance of the tree or the imagery for face value. There is usually opportunity to return to an image or to revisit when the therapeutic alliance has developed further. It can be difficult to process in the realm of symbols, but I love it when a client begins to find their own symbolic language and world of metaphors. This liminal space is ripe for movement, growth, repair, and transition.

Working with Opposites and the Space in Between: Directives

In order to help move into symbols and metaphor and ultimately the creative levels, I think working with the space in between opposites and juxtapositions can be helpful. There are a number of directives that are helpful with this, but there are also a number of ways that are more focused on materials versus directives. I enjoy the materials-based exploration the most, but that being said, the directives are excellent introductory forays into this world if a client or a therapist is unaccustomed to moving into this space.

Creating connection and space between opposing forces can be helpful and illuminating. For example, I was teaching a Psychopathology course and was finding that there was a disconnect for graduate students between the diagnostic process ("labeling") and healing/repair. I asked the students to fold a piece of paper into three spaces; on the left, I asked them to draw their feelings about diagnosis. On the right side, I asked them to draw what healing and repair looked like to them. In the center, I asked them to find a way to connect the two images that felt authentic to them. What happened was an embodied sense to increase discernment around diagnosis versus rejection or dismissal; of course, not every student became magically enthralled by the idea of diagnosis, but there was an ability to at least consider the positive aspects of having a common language to coordinate treatment planning and to communicate with multidisciplinary teams.

For clients, I find that the "a better day/not as great day" directive can be a good start. I stay away from the words "bad" and "good" as a day is not entirely bad or entirely good in essence. It can also limit a client, but with little ones, good and bad might make the most sense. With this, I ask that the client paint, draw, or sculpt their response and then consider the ways that the less positive day could become more positive and vice versa. I have also used the problem/solution juxtaposition and then what the magic wand could provide to move the problem closer to the solution. Returning to the emotions directive mentioned previously, we can pick two emotions that are somewhat opposing and then work on connecting these to the body. Turning one over and feeling the impact in the body and then repeating the action with the other drawing can be helpful to notice somatically what happens in the body when both emotions are visible versus just one or the other. Taking these emotions and exploring where they live in the body can be helpful with addressing somatic issues and "growing" the positive into the less pleasant emotional spaces offers space for repair.

Conversely, I may begin with the somatic space and then move into the artwork depending on client readiness. I will ask a client where they are noting any looseness or sense of calm/happiness, etc., in the body. Sometimes a positive sensation may be difficult to identify; if so, the less pleasant sensation may be easier to identify. Many of my clients experience chronic pain or a chronic health condition that correlates to cumulative trauma; I myself deal with chronic migraines, and on days of pain, it may be difficult to recognize that there is anywhere in the body that actually feels good or isn't directly impacted by the pain. I will ask the client to try to attach a color, texture, temperature, or any other sensory element to the more pleasant sensation and then to do the same with the less pleasant or painful place (or vice versa). I painted my representation of calm and peacefulness that I could access in my body in the first image. In the second image, I created what the pain was looking like in my head. There was a distinct difference in temperature noted in the color choices as well as the texture; the first image is cool and smooth with small waves, while the second was hot, spiky, and full of nervousness/anxiety (Figures 10.1 and 10.2).

I then considered for myself, and we often do this in session, which 3D materials in the room could represent the 2D imagery. I chose a heavy rock on a piece of cool blue paper and a spiky red ball that I really disliked the texture of in my hands. Moving between exploring and feeling the differences in weight, solidity, texture, color, etc., and then allowing the body to choose

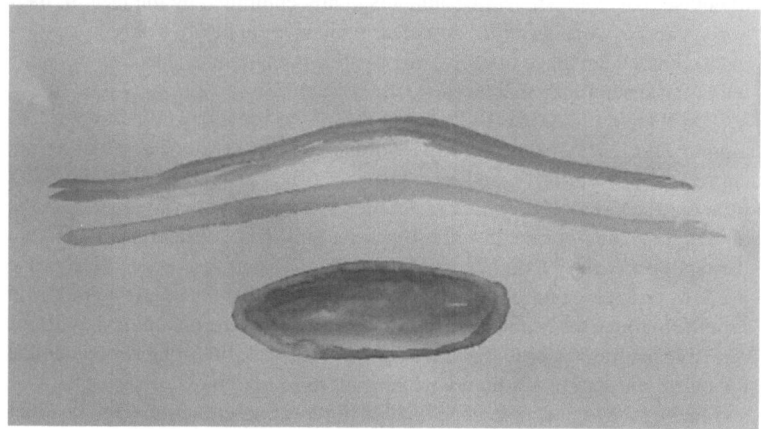

Figure 10.1 Image of calm created by the author.

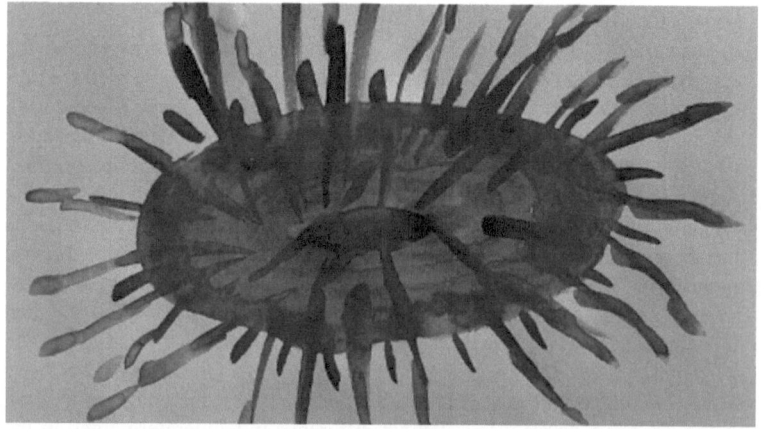

Figure 10.2 Image of anxiety created by the author.

how it wants to respond or what it would like to do next can be useful. What I noticed for myself and what I witness or co-experience with clients is a shift from the emphasis on the painful to a movement toward the less painful or the more healing/regulating. The next step is to consider what the symbols/emotions may be connected to in current life experiences and ways to increase the positive sensations or at least avoid/decrease some of the areas of life that exacerbate pain or even fight, flight, and freeze responses. For myself, I noted that the pain correlated to fight, flight, and freeze in my image and that if I could stay in my window of tolerance, the pain became less intense. Creating movement and oscillation or pendulation between the opposites increases the ability to move between the states and to connect more intentionally to the more positive sensations. Walking between the two symbols or turning them over, moving the 3D representations between the hands helps with bilateral connection. Being able to re-experience positive options and find the body as a resource as opposed to an enemy may alleviate some aspects of mental health symptomology. It is essential as trauma survivors that we can remember that the body can protect us and hold reparative sensations and feelings instead of simply traumatic experiences. Being able to tolerate a tiptoe into less pleasant sensations in the context of a resource helps to build confidence and to decrease fight, flight, freeze, and fawn responses.

Working with opposites and the space in between can be done with almost any type of juxtaposition and an intervention that can be tailor-made for a client spontaneously in session. Adolescents sometimes come into sessions with uncertainty around body image or their external presentation. We may create imagery around some of areas of the body or their appearance that they appreciate and then some of the areas that are less embraced; I will then ask them to connect these in some way or to consider if there are any parts that are more neutral that we could use to increase the positivity or to create affirmations around. When clients are trying to make decisions, it can be useful to use the two sides of the decision and then create the space in between the poles, represented in art form. Being able to utilize symbol and metaphor to represent the opposing elements can offer a different viewpoint as well as a more embodied and creative way to garner resolution and to close a loop or at least to encourage further exploration.

Working with Opposites and the Space in Between: Materials

In my office, I have a leaning tower of boxes of all shapes and sizes from small papier-mâché boxes to shoe boxes to cigar boxes (sometimes it takes some airing out to get the smell of cigars out of these) to larger packing boxes. My husband laughs at me because we seem to never leave a garage sale or a flea market without an armful of containers. Boxes implicitly offer containment, multiple surfaces, and an inside and an outside. They can become transitional objects; they can hold things. Clearly, I can't say enough good things about boxes in art therapy, but I think that their easy melding into a creative space for symbology and metaphor making as well as the potential to be aesthetically pleasing and intrinsically useful makes them appealing for clients.

Directives are easy to use with boxes such as inside/outside boxes where a client creates what they hold for themselves on the inside of the box and what they choose to show to the world on the outside. However, I like to let the box progression take shape for a client to develop for themselves. Just offering choice and then allowing the direction to be spontaneous seems to be most conducive to allowing a client to engage in their own symbolic language and metaphor. With little ones, I remember stories of outer space, video game worlds, intricate landscapes with a variety of creatures, etc., that came to life utilizing the inside and the outside of the boxes for storytelling and for the expression of uncontrollable real-life situations that felt less terrifying in the containment of the box through symbolic representation. Boxes also offer a space for play and for interaction if the figures are moveable and interchangeable. I also had a client create a life-size favorite wrestler out of boxes that had the power and the physical control that the individual wanted to have for himself but could not due to a physical disability; being able to create a life-size human lent a sense of mastery. The wrestler was the mascot for the art therapy space for quite some time, greeted each week by the kiddo with a playful high five.

Sometimes the boxes become an outlet to safely place things that feel intolerable in a literal sense. While decorating the outside of a box, a client decided to make symbols of her deepest darkest secrets that were coded so that she would only understand them; these secrets were causing the client to engage in "morbid reflection" and shame to a point that she remained in a cycle of self-harm and substance use to numb the impact of the shame. She wanted to put the slips of paper with the symbols of the secrets in the box and asked to leave the box at my office; we locked it in a drawer of my filing cabinet. Several weeks later, I asked about the box and the slips of paper; she stated that she had forgotten about it altogether. She also had had no instances of self-harm and was not using substances; we talked about the connection of allowing someone else to hold the secrets for her in a safe space. It was not important that I know the secrets but just that the secrets were out of her body and securely tucked away where no one had to know what they were. Eventually, we had a ceremony where we burned the box and the secrets in a safe way outdoors.

Multiple clients have created imagery of the things that they like about themselves and things that they like in general on the outside of the box. Often the inside holds things that the client may feel less positive about, connected to, or attached to about themselves. We have taken time to create positive affirmations either through art pieces or through written slips of paper that get placed inside the box to help ease the impact of the areas and to decrease their power. We take time to place the papers or pieces into the box intentionally and note what the somatic sensation is as each item goes into the box. This continues to connect and reconnect to the body, the emotions, and the spirit; as the process continues, we evaluate emotional regulation and sensory integration in conjunction with the cognitive/symbolic levels, abstract thinking, and executive function. The idea that all art in some way is a self-portrait of the creator may or may not have merit, but when working with the dichotomy of an inside and an outside, whether it be a box or a different container, and altered book or a terrarium, etc., there is a felt sense of this.

Personal Symbols and Social Atoms

Embarking upon symbol creation, sometimes card decks, sand play, or work with model magic or clay can be helpful. Utilizing Krans' *The Wild Unknown Animal Spirit Deck and Guidebook* can be a playful and often powerful approach. Having a client draw a card and then consider the qualities of the animal that they drew, connecting this to themselves in some way, is a nice entry point to moving into the symbolic. The book gives a brief description of the qualities of the animal, what brings these qualities into balance and what can make them out of balance as well as the gifts that the animal spirit holds. This can jump-start a rich conversation about the client's own qualities, how they relate or don't relate to the animal spirit, and what helps them be in balance versus what throws them off track. From this discussion, the client can respond with an art response, movement, or writing to reflect. This can be useful in family, individual, or group work to help people understand what is support for them versus what tends to be triggering or discombobulating. Being able to pendulate between talking about self and talking about an animal spirit allows for movement between the metaphorical/symbolic and the self, creating a safety and feeling of objectivity/distance between the self and the animal where the client has the ability to choose how intimate or how removed they want to be in the process.

We tend to work with symbols implicitly; the work of the art therapist is to make the implicit or what lies in the shadow realm come to the surface with intentionality and with support. All art has purpose and holds multiple layers of meaning that reveal themselves over time and through supportive reflection and conversation. For example, during a recent professional seminar course, it is my practice to paint alongside students in the response painting process we utilize for art therapy supervision. The intention is to provide a container and expressive response to client and clinical work throughout the term utilizing a process painting procedure. The only requirements are to utilize a surface that is 24″ × 36″ or larger and to paint weekly during our class referencing their client interactions/internship experiences over the previous week. The painting I created during this term was of two snails under a full moon, framed and sheltered by two weeping willows. Throughout the term, there were moments of heaviness and joy, of overwhelm and fatigue in tandem with joy and with "therapeutic wins." I noted my own need as well as the needs of students to allow a trust in the process and to slow down, to move more intentionally noting that they were leaving an impact on clients and on their internship sites much like the trail a snail leaves upon every surface they climb across. I considered the parallel processes of the two snails, though they were going in different directions; this seemed to mirror instructor to student, supervisor to student, student to client, people to people. I could feel the shadow self moving with the known self in a slow and careful dance as each reveals themselves to one another while being witnessed by the moon and sheltered by the trees. When I began the image, all I knew is that I wanted a dark background and a hill; the rest came forward from week to week with gradual revelations. I am aware that more will be revealed in time. My students had different thoughts and reflections, which made the experience richer and deeper. Personal symbology can be a gradual unfolding and development, or it can be deliberate and known from the onset (Figure 10.3).

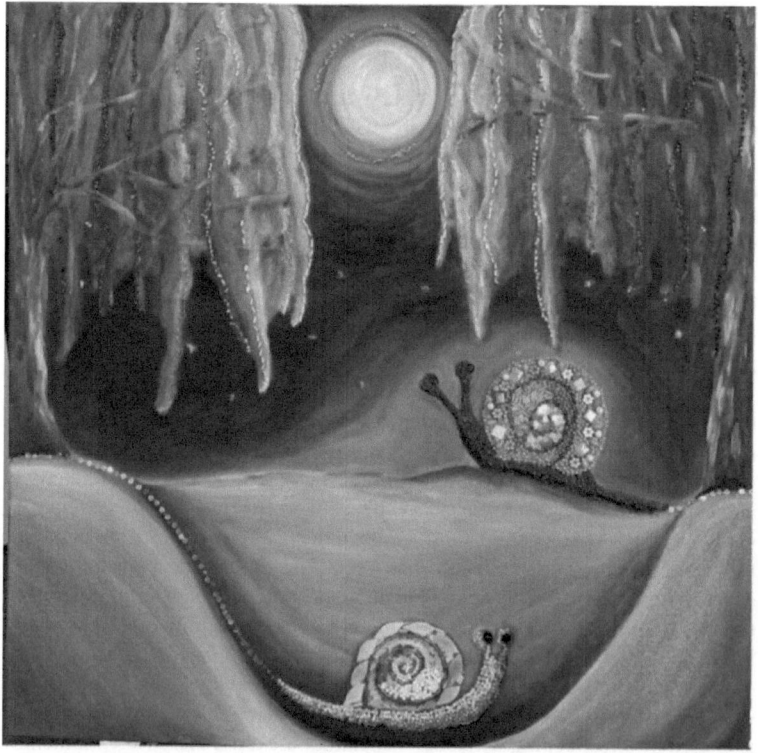

Figure 10.3 Snail imagery created by the author; oil paint on canvas with mixed media.

There are several directives that can be useful to assist clients with moving into the symbolic/metaphorical level. I might offer a client several mask form options, ranging from animal to blank face to magical being. From here, I ask them to complete both the outside and the inside of the mask, playing with the opposites of the part that looks inward toward them versus what faces the outside world. We can dialogue between the two sides or gain a somatic understanding of how the inside of the mask feels versus the outside, how these sides communicate with the outside world or the inner dialogue. Otherwise, we can create a mask together with papier-mâché, cardboard, tissue paper, embellishments, etc. Donning a mask allows us to see ourselves in a different light or to try on an identity perhaps that we wish we had; superheroes (and sometimes the antihero), warriors, and fantastical beings are popular subject matter. Frida Kahlo stated that she made self-portraits because she was solitary with herself much of the time; I've also heard the statement from a dear friend: "I may not be much, but I'm all I ever think about." As people, self-introspection can turn into perseverance or rumination, even obsession, but in healthy doses, we need to spend time with self-representation in order to explore and to repair ourselves. Seeing ourselves from a number of different symbolic angles and perspectives presents the ability to gain a more objective sense of self and to be able to view ourselves perhaps as people who love us might see us so that we can learn to do this for ourselves. Being able to step into a sense of personal power and greater autonomy can be useful with repair.

Another directive working with symbols is utilizing a social atom. Tian Dayton is an expert on social atoms and sociometry in the framework of relational trauma repair and psychodrama. I have adapted Dayton's model of the social atom to an art therapy intervention but have also used Dayton's model of processing in groupwork. Her website (https://www.tiandayton.com), videos, and books have a multitude of excellent resources. When using the social atom, I will ask a client to draw a personal symbol for themselves in the center of the page and then drawing a circle around the symbol; from here, I will ask them to draw symbols of people, places, things, animals, and institutions that have important associations in their life, whether those be positive, distant, or what they perceive as negative. I have asked people to create two social atoms if it feels beneficial to have the person create the atom considering where they wish all of these items were in relation to themselves and then another page where they consider where the items are in relation to their personal symbol currently. Often pets or the closest of people can be in the inner circle or very close in proximity; we then explore the relational ties between the personal symbol and the additional objects, creating lines that depict the type of relationships. For example, if it is an "on again/off again" relationship, the line may be dotted. If the client's energy goes toward the person but they don't feel like they receive much in return, it may be an arrow going from the client toward the other person's symbol. These relational lines can show strong bonds or conflict; this is particularly helpful with individuals who may be having the majority of the relationships online as this can be depicted with monitors or with internet cables, etc. If desired, this can be done in a sand tray, with props and puppets, or on paper cut outs (collage, drawn, etc.) where the individual can move the different people, places, animals, and things to test out how it feels to have the relationships become closer or more distant. What people choose to represent themselves as well as to represent relevant players in their lives are valuable areas of information; this intervention can be useful with addiction recovery to identify ruptures, areas of present day to leave behind, and new people and places that could be supportive in the journey forward. This practice allows the ability to zoom in and to zoom out, to have magic moments and then create practical steps to try to make wishes more attainable, and to analyze areas that could be unhealthy or possibly abusive. In the photo, there is a sand play example of a social atom in sand and with figurines. The bird houses and bird in the center represent the individual's different worlds and relationships depicted through the different areas delineated in the sand tray. There is a cemetery in the corner that holds a departed caregiver; school is the lighthouse and apple tree. The koi pond is where an individual would like to spend more time in a home that doesn't exist for them yet; the central area of bird houses is anchored by fairies and mythical creatures that are guarding the individual. Potentially, there could be an opening to connect these creatures to areas of self or to key people who exist in current reality. Whether processing is verbal or somatic in nature, the metaphors that are created can translate into real-world application when examining resiliency factors and resources (Figure 10.4).

In art therapy, there are a multitude of ways to engage the cognitive, symbolic, and metaphorical levels of the ETC and to connect/bridge the sensory

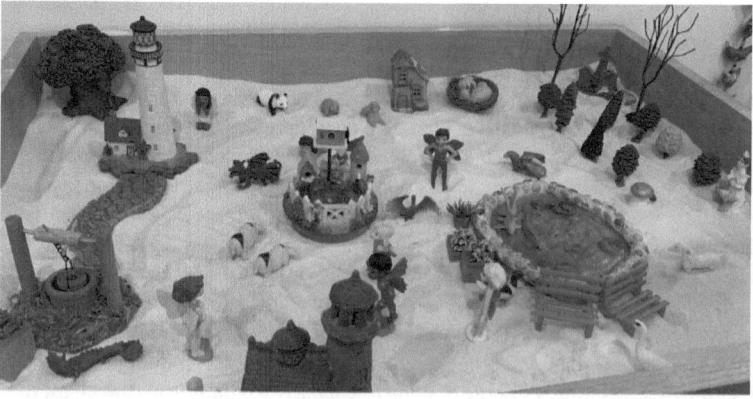

Figure 10.4 Sand play image created by the author for the purpose of illustrating this concept.

and the emotional realms with executive functioning. This chapter has delved into a few, but any time the somatic areas are brought into areas of emotional expression, the sensory and the relational, the creative level can come forward. These are those "aha" moments or the times where you can visibly observe a person experience a shift away from rupture and into safety and repair. When an active sense of safety and operating within the optimal arousal zone is achieved, creativity and imagination can be explored and engaged.

References

Hinz, L.D., Rim, S., & Lusebrink, V. B. (2022). Clarifying the creative level of the expressive therapies continuum: A different dimension. *The Arts in Psychotherapy,* Volume 78, April 2022. https://doi.org/10.1016/j.aip.2022.101896

Taylor-Johnson, H. (2023). Knitting as a way of honoring Black ancestry and creating storytelling through community, belonging, and the reframing of grief: A womanist perspective. *Canadian Journal of Art Therapy, 36*(1), 12–19. https://doi.org/10.108 0/26907240.2023.2199623

11 The Creative and the Imagination Network

Have you ever been in an act of creation (painting, drawing, working with mixed media, etc.) and recognized that hours have passed with no other thoughts, interruptions, or concerns except for the art process? The colors feel right in your body. Somewhere in that process, was there an "I got this" feeling or a mental and/or physical hopping up and down with glee regarding pleasure in the process and in the product's emergence? There is a connection between what has been termed a "flow state" (Csíkmentmihálhyi, 1996) and positive self-regard, increased positive feelings. I have experienced this flow state in the therapeutic realm when a client and therapist have a synergistic rhythmic healing process; like a flow state, sometimes this is easier to achieve or to tap into than other times. As mentioned in prior chapters, it is necessary for the other areas of the Expressive Therapies Continuum (ETC) and Neurosequential Model of Therapeutics' four functional domains to be in balance to engage in the flow.

Resiliency and a sense of safety are necessary components. In addition, there is a sense that perhaps something larger is happening aside from just human connection in this intersubjectivity. When the creative realm is entered, for those of us who lean into a spiritual aspect of our work and/or for our clients who have a spiritual practice, it may be helpful to consider that there is a large universal beneficence at play, a spiritual dimension of sorts that supports and fosters creativity. I have highly valued the Second Step in Alcoholics Anonymous for my own recovery process: "Came to believe that a Power greater than ourselves could restore us to sanity" (p. 59). The sanity that is described relates to being free from an addictive substance and return to our true selves without this substance. A spiritual connection is recommended, but this is a higher power of your own choosing, selection, or construction. Being open as clinicians to the spiritual realm and being culturally responsive, curious, and supportive of our client's spiritual beliefs can pave a pathway to the imaginal and creative realm.

Whyte (2023) couches the ETC in the context of spirituality, defining the spirit/creative dimension as "the energy of determination…the energy that brings us to our gifts and life path. This is where creativity and flow thrive

DOI: 10.4324/9781032695228-16

because the energy is connected with the beauty of the self" (p. 2). Linking spirit with the creative dimension of the continuum, this section of the circle can be described as the fluid movement across the continuum and deep engagement in the material process. Through engagement with the creative and spiritual dimension, there is the possibility to "develop new skills, engage in self-reflection, and develop new views of the self and the world. In turn, through the integration of increased competence, new self-knowledge, and novel insights individual resilience is strengthened" (p. 2). This center meeting point for all levels of the ETC creates a nexus for the creative and the spiritual, which can be felt somatically, spiritually, and emotionally.

With spirituality and creativity, there is the necessary reinstatement of a sense of safety and resiliency by beginning at the kinesthetic/sensory level and working up to the cognitive and creative levels. Resiliency is the ability to overcome potential negative effects and symptoms from events that would otherwise cause negative outcomes; creative imagery is a way to increase resiliency (Rak & Patterson, 1996, p. 371). Play and imagination are essential for resiliency. When survival is the predominant goal, trauma can render a child and/or adult unable to play or to tap into the imagination (Streeck-Fischer & van der Kolk, 2000). "Play is a powerful stimulant for organizing a brain that fosters the creation of joy, curiosity, and exploration" (Kravits, 2008, p. 139). Individuals who become accustomed to operating out of a survival perspective struggle with fantasy and symbolization. Art therapy can begin the process of reawakening the capacity for the higher-level functions of fantasy and symbolization by first approaching the sensory and somatic aspects on the bottom-up level. Chong (2015) wrote,

Art materials offer a unique capacity to absorb and slow down high impulse emotions. The ability to slow down high impulse emotions is a big leap in opening up opportunities for the cortex to be reconnected, and thus to get involved in the process of stress response.

(p. 122)

To address the spectrum of trauma responses, it is essential to reduce impulsivity and to increase response time, creating a longer period of felt safety.

Pointon (2004) stated that there is a power through the drawing process, which is "an activity that re-engages the prefrontal cortex of the brain and provides an alternative way of symbolically representing trauma" (p. 5). This has the potential to restore that lost capacity for imagination. Siegel and Hartzell (2004) called the higher parts of the brain, or the neocortex, and their integration with the lower regions of the brain, or the brain stem, the "high road." The "low road" tends to be void of higher processing abilities such as self-reflection, attunement, and empathy. Traumatized individuals respond to stimuli with the low road much more quickly. When triggers are apparent, the reactions are exaggerated and harder to extinguish.

Art therapists, Hass-Cohen and Carr (2008), discussed the high road versus the low road as well. They discussed how survival responses emerge from the low road, arousing the sympathetic nervous system. For the high road, there is a complete circuit of the brain, involving all portions and integrating the different sections, allowing for decision-making and greater awareness to occur. For children who have experienced trauma, impulsivity and anger management issues are common. "Sensory art therapy practices stimulate thalamic connections to and from cortical and subcortical brain regions. ... Sensory enriched, multi-modal, self- and other-regulated environments are known to help 'bottom-up' and 'top-down' approaches coordinate and deregulate thalamic gateway functions" (2008, p. 50).

Streeck-Fischer and van der Kolk (2000) emphasized the need for a mediator between inner and outer reality that can provide a space and relationship that is conducive for fantasy and creativity. This connects to the previous discussion regarding containers; the mediator may be the artwork itself; it may be the intersubjective space between the art, the clinician, and the client(s), or potentially the mediator may be a universal or spiritual support for the therapy process. Considering best options for moving into the imaginal realm, there are numerous pathways into this arena, both directive and nondirective. If working in a family system or a group, or even exploring relationship between therapist and client, the kingdom intervention (Schroder, 2004, p. 25) offers a structured imaginal exploration. The participants are given a large sheet of paper with a section created for each individual; the instruction is that they have been gifted a kingdom and can draw anything that they would like in their section utilizing an array of drawing materials. After the completion of this step, the participants are asked if they would like to connect the kingdoms in some way, leaving this a choice to connect or the ability to set a firm boundary. Interestingly enough, when I have utilized this in session, I find that people tend to allow themselves to move into the imaginal realm with the idea of being gifted a kingdom. It seems to be a direct connection to fantasy and to personal world construction. There is a container and the possibility for boundary exploration in an imaginal and creative realm.

In a similar vein, Gavron's Joint Painting Procedure (2013) creates containment with the possibility for connection. I have adapted this procedure so that it can completed between therapist and client, client and other participant(s), a group, etc., though Gavron's intention was for the traditional assessment to be dyadic. The first step is to mark personal space on a large piece of paper in pencil; then, the space can be filled in with paint in any manner the participant selects. Then a frame is created around the personal space; if desired, the participants can create a path between their own framed piece to the other pieces created. Gavron then suggests a fifth step where the participants paint together in a joint area without changing their personal areas of pathways. When this is completed in session, depending on how the participants are feeling somatically, they can decide as to whether or not they would like to complete the fifth step (it also depends on if connection was formed in the fourth step).

This is beneficial since this procedure creates the possibility for alignment between group members, therapist and client, family systems, etc., but most importantly, it allows for an individual, autonomous imaginal process within a container of their own creation that can be shared or held to themselves. This could also be done on separate sheets of paper with the decision made between participants as to whether a connection is desired to allow for more individual creative space. With the client creating their own metaphorical space and framework to engage in creativity, it may bring a somatic aware-ness and symbolic representation that it is possible for the client to do this for themselves in their worlds outside of the therapeutic milieu.

The superhero directive is simply to draw yourself as a superhero. This can be challenging for individuals who have experienced trauma due to possible feelings of powerlessness. It can be a foray into power exploration and an ability to step into power and control on an imaginal and metaphorical level. I remember offering this to a young boy in the foster system with complex trauma systems; rather than drawing this, he asked me if I would help him create a cape. We did this with tissue paper, pieces of cloth, a stapler, and Velcro strips as this was impromptu; on the cape, we worked together to in-clude the client's superpowers and the different elements in his life that kept him strong. He donned the cape and ran around the office, showing this off for his family and explaining how he wanted to use his powers. With adults, this imagery may feel more subtle, but allowing adults to return to stories of their favorite superheroes, cartoons, video games, movies, etc., and then to the art process promotes movement into forces of good and evil, ways that they can use their superpowers in their own lives. In addition, we can explore the superhero's "kryptonite," alter ego, personal mission, etc. Expanding on this idea, I offered a group of teenage boys in an after-school program bins full of recycled materials. With these materials, I asked them to create a city and to work together. They initially created their own buildings, vehicles, people, animals, etc., with these materials, even making miniature billboards and traf-fic lights. With a little support, they were able to then decide how to put these elements together and to play together, moving into the spaces that they had created. This was a major feat given previous displays of territorialism with art supplies due to heightened survival instincts and hypervigilance stemming from cumulative trauma. Watching the play and the connection happening was surprising. We were all down on the ground making car sounds and en-gaging in pretending, imaginal play.

Fairy tales can offer a foray into the imaginal realm; changing the ending or components of an existing fairy tale, creating one's own, writing the tale in partnership, or even shifting the narrative of one's own personal story to have different endings or fantasy elements can be healing and restorative. Pretending to have a crystal ball and to create what is seen in the crystal ball can give fertile ground for future hopes and dreams. Offering a magic wand solution to dream of, even momentarily, can offer space to consider different options.

Beginning with directives initially helps to reconnect individuals with the imagination or with the possibility of accessing imagination, creativity, and joy independently without the aid of the therapeutic container. I provide journals for clients to use outside of session to draw, collage, paint, or draw. Clients who previously did not have an art or writing practice will come into session showing me digital art or projects that they have embarked upon at home. I had a client who also maintained an "art therapy closet" where they put up all of their art from our sessions so that they could go and sit with their pieces without disturbance from pets and children. They told me that they had moments of calm in this closet, surrounded by their imagery. When moving into working with creativity without directives, offering a wide array of materials and options will give greater freedom and engagement into imagination, play, and joy. If having "too much choice" feels like a barrier, offering choice between two and three items at a time and whittling down until an idea is grasped are ideal. Being able to operate in the proverbial "sweet spot" of art therapy is a rewarding and joyous place to share with clients as a therapist, collaborator, and witness.

References

Chong, C. Y. J. (2015). Why art psychotherapy? Through the lens of interpersonal neurobiology: The distinctive role of art psychotherapy intervention for clients with early relational trauma. *International Journal of Art Therapy, 20*(3), 118–126. https://doi.org/10.1080/17454832.2015.1079727

Csíkmentmihálhyi, M. (1996). *Creativity: Flow and the psychology of discovery and invention.* New York: Harper Collins.

Gavron, T. (2013). Meeting on common ground: Assessing parent–child relationships through the Joint Painting Procedure. *Art Therapy, 30*(1), 12–19. https://doi.org/10.1080/07421656.2013.757508

Hass-Cohen, N., & Carr, R. (2008). *Art therapy and clinical neuroscience.* London: Jessica Kingsley.

Kravits, K. (2008). The neurobiology of relatedness: Attachment. In N. Hass-Cohen & R. Carr (Eds.), *Art therapy and clinical neuroscience* (pp. 131–146). London: Jessica Kingsley.

Pointon, C. (2004). The future of trauma work. *Counseling and Psychotherapy Journal, 14*(4), 3–10.

Rak, C. F., & Patterson, L. E. (1996). Promoting resilience in at-risk children. *Journal of Counseling & Development, 74*(4), 368–373. https://doi.org/10.1002/j.1556-6676.1996.tb01881

Schroder, D. (2004). *Little windows into art therapy: Small openings for beginning art therapists.* Philadelphia, PA: Jessica Kingsley Publishers.

Siegel, D., & Hartzell, M. (2004). *Parenting from the inside out.* New York: Penguin.

Streeck-Fischer, A., & van der Kolk, B. A. (2000). Down will come baby, cradle and all: Diagnostic and therapeutic implications of chronic trauma on child development. *Australian and New Zealand Journal of Psychiatry, 34,* 903–918. https://doi.org/10.1080/000486700265

Whyte, M. K. (2023). Stepping into the circle: Inviting spirit through medicine wheel teachings in the expressive therapies Continuum. *Canadian Journal of Art Therapy, 36*(1), 20–30. https://doi.org/10.1080/26907240.2023.2210984

12 Survival Responses and Adaptive Options

Perry (personal communication, April 6, 2015) stated that by using the neurosequential assessment, treatment teams could "quantify developmental adversity vs. resilience-related factors." Resilience-related factors include support people, coping strategies, optimism, talents, and so forth. These factors act as buffers that decrease the impact of the developmental adversity. If an individual has minimal support and few coping mechanisms, then exposure to traumatic events has greater effects. This results in a decreased level of executive functioning, creating the perfect candidate for art therapy and nonverbal strategies (B. D. Perry, personal communication, April 6, 2015). The assessment lens of the Neurosequential Model of Therapeutics (NMT) focuses on key facets such as demographics; history (developmental, adverse events measure, and relational health measure); current status (central nervous system functional status measure and relational health measure); and recommendations made for the therapeutic web, the family, and the client. There are four areas that are focused on for the client: sensory integration and self-regulation. The NMT assessment is a way of creating a map for educators, caregivers, clients, and the therapeutic web. The NMT assessment lens provides clear-cut indications to which interventions will be the most efficient and appropriate.

As mentioned in prior chapters and in alignment with the Expressive Therapies Continuum, the first entry point is to address "bottom-up somatosensory regulatory routes" where rhythmic and repetitive activities can calm "neural networks that originate in the lower parts of the brain and are essential to the stress response" (MacKinnon, 2012, p. 215). There are many art therapy interventions that are able to provide the rhythm and repetition that are indicated through the NMT model utilizing clay and tactile materials, scribble drawings, the acts of painting and drawing or coloring, papier-mâché, newspaper sculptures, and other options. In my experience in treating trauma symptoms in dysregulated youth, I begin by providing tactile options such as clay or Play-Doh, coloring materials, and so on. I often suggest sitting on the ground and using repetitive motions to knead the clay or Play-Doh or to color. The

DOI: 10.4324/9781032695228-17

motions usually begin as chaotic and fast until the client's body begins to regulate. The autonomic nervous system comes back online and into a rhythm that assists with an overall grounding process.

Dissociation in a controlled fashion also can be regulatory in the forms of daydreaming, doodling, and distraction. By engaging the bottom-up processes, the top-down systems can begin to operate and interact on a developmentally appropriate level. By doing so, the cortex will eventually mature, strengthening in functioning. "The maturation and strengthening of the cortex occurs through mastering the bottom-up and then introducing the addition of the acquisition of language, interacting in social situations, and other top-down processes" (MacKinnon, 2012, p. 215).

Outpatient therapy and higher levels of care can be integral to jump-starting a reduction in survival responses such as fight, flight, freeze, submit, and/or attach; however, more regular practice of coping strategies, an increase in resiliency and support factors, and an integration of replacement behavioral options are needed outside of the therapeutic milieu. Perry's therapeutic web suggests a multidisciplinary team that can potentially offer music therapy, physical and/or occupational therapy, art therapy, psychiatric care (if applicable), support people, family and friends, etc., who can offer multiple avenues into repair and healing. Due to socioeconomic and systemic barriers, this may not be an option. I find that I must be creative and be able to improvise to fit the client's needs and to adapt to available resources.

Substance use, process addictions, disordered eating, self-harm, and other maladaptive patterns are survival strategies that have outlived their welcome for many trauma survivors including myself. The need to find other options to satisfy the holes that are left when these practices are discontinued becomes urgent and essential. I had a sense of shame for using substances, food, perfectionism, overwork, and relationships to decrease hypervigilance, dissociation, and anxiety. Each adaptive attempt had its benefits and drawbacks; I began to develop greater self-compassion from recognizing that these were my best efforts toward self-healing and self-medication. When I learned that these attempts were killing me instead of healing me, I came to the place that I witness in many of my clients. Knowing is one thing; repairing and healing is another. Finding healthier replacement options was key until I had the stability and the foundation to operate from my optimal arousal zone and with proper support options and processes.

From my own experiences and with supporting individuals in clinical practice, there are ways to create an "ad hoc" therapeutic web that can be effective and cost-efficient considering access to transportation, stage of change, and personal time limitations. Community support groups are often free or low cost and can offer a sense of belonging, a reduction in "uniqueness," and a structured approach to relationship development and coping strategies. Most offer virtual options or multiple times that fit work, parenting, and school schedules. Many provide peer mentorship or sponsorship where a member slightly further along can support a newcomer. Discerning whether there are family members or friends who could come into the therapeutic milieu and learn ways to support the client can be a possibility.

Besides support options, there are many at-home practices that can be replacement possibilities for addictive patterns. I integrate daily art options and journal practice. The altered book process can be excellent for home; the "Wreck This Journal" series (Smith, 2012) is fun and a great way to start a daily art practice that reduces perfectionism or paralysis and procrastination due to perfectionism. I had a client who maintained a "scribble journal" for over a year where she scribbled in the book daily until her body told her that she was done. We reviewed the journal each week and discussed the somatic responses that she logged in tandem with the scribbles. Working with small body maps to identify areas of positivity and areas of pain can be useful. This gives clients the option to track shifts over time regarding chronic pain and efficacy of coping strategies, considering each day based on the map what the body may need. Utilizing apps on devices for check-ins in the morning and at night can be helpful and provide better tracking in between sessions and more emotional expression daily rather than processing solely during the session time. With these different processes, there is a slight structure and a container that offer flexibility and creativity; this extends a sense of account-ability and dedication to the therapeutic and repair process while simultane-ously generating healthier coping options and increasing self-awareness and self-reflexivity.

It is essential to remember what you used to like, what used to inspire you, and even what you wanted to be when you grew up. I utilize interest inven-tories and collage practice to discern likes and dislikes that can be forgotten while in survival mode and/or addictive patterns. Reconnecting with hopes and dreams and selecting snippets of these that can be revisited can reinvigor-ate motivation and future planning. Creating treatment plans that offer move-ment toward these hopes and dreams in practical, expressive, and enjoyable ways can be reparative and enjoyable. I have clients who now garden and tell stories of a yearning toward this in childhood or a sweet moment with a trusted adult helping in the garden that now can be revisited when their hands touch the soil. Cooking, making music, dancing to music, and singing are all amazing options; if those feel too big, it may simply be moving from the couch to sit closer to a window and feel sun on your face or watch the rain/snow fall. There is no coping strategy too small; I think when I first started in practice, I had an incorrect idea that treatment plans needed to feel bigger and that steps to meet goals needed to be more sizeable. This was not considerate or clinically beneficial. It can be overwhelming or discouraging to be told that what you already doing for your own health isn't enough or that you don't know what is best for you. Client's hold their own medicine; my role is simply to reacquaint them with their own healing capabilities. Being able to support clients where they are and to expand on what they are already implementing may be what is best. Offering positive feedback and encouragement for planting seeds and giving the safety and the compassionate space for the seeds to grow seem to be the best practice.

References

MacKinnon, L. (2012). The neurosequential model of therapeutics: An interview with Bruce Perry. *The Australian & New Zealand Journal of Family Therapy, 33*(3), 210–218. Doi:10.1017/aft.2012.26

Smith, K. (2012). *Wreck This Journal.* New York: Penguin Books.

Perry, B.D., personal communication, April 6, 2015.

Part VI

Conclusion

"In the haunted house of life, art is the only stair that doesn't creak" (Robbins, 2003, p. 37).

When I began the doctorate process in art therapy, it began as a way to perfect my "art therapy and trauma repair" elevator speech. I was exhausted from attempting to explain what I was seeing in practice that was working; I was frustrated by being told that this interconnection between art therapy and neurobiology, bottom-up and top-down, expressive and cognitive processes was not "evidence-based." I wanted to have the words and the research behind me to feel confident in my clinical practice and in a felt sense that repair was happening in the therapeutic realm. I wanted to be able to answer the question that Klorer (2005) posed: "How does this work?" (p. 218), when referring to the effectiveness of art therapy interventions in healing trauma wounds. I knew what had worked in my own ongoing reparative healing, and I have had over 20 years of clinical practice in an array of therapeutic venues. Throughout this journey, the bridge between art therapy and trauma repair has been essential in all aspects of clinical practice. Though the art therapy field has understood on an implicit level that art therapy appears to be effective for treating trauma, pairing neuroscience with art therapy assists in providing evidence-based explanations as to how this works. This explanation is important for other medical professionals, caregivers, educators, and others to get a sense of how art therapy works with trauma repair. This has been helpful in honing the proverbial elevator speech.

In addition, if other helping professionals do not have further understanding regarding the need for nonverbal interventions, clients may continue to be inaccurately diagnosed and/or treated. Gantt and Tinnin (2009) suggested that this is not a time to delay treatment or to conclude that a client is not compliant with treatment simply because a client cannot discuss the trauma on a top-down level.

Art therapy is effective for trauma survivors not because it bypasses defenses but because it provides a path where none existed previously.

DOI:10.4324/9781032695228-18

If peritraumatic dissociation disrupts the coding of experience in words, memories are still laid down but in the nonverbal part of the brain.

(Gantt & Tinnin, 2009, p. 151)

Traumatic memories are not stored in the brain in the same way that autobiographical memories are. These memories are tied to the nonverbal; they are coded as emotional and sensory experiences. These memories may be intrusive and involve physical sensations and emotions. The sensations tend to be visual in nature but may also be connected to sounds, smells, and textures.

Retrieval is not the most important component of trauma treatment. In fact, what is felt implicitly may not be retrievable in a verbal or cognitive sense. What is most important is to be able to integrate traumatic memories and to begin addressing the effects of implicit memories. Talwar (2007) stated that the "integration of traumatic experiences is dependent upon the bilateral stimulation of the frontal lobes. … Non-verbal expressive therapies … all activate the subcortical regions" (p. 26). This integration is essential to reduce the survival responses that may occur without a clear trigger or source. Without integration, it is nearly impossible to decrease hypervigilance and/or dissociation. This feels important to emphasize given the continued emphasis on exposure and a reliance on executive functioning in trauma treatment versus a creative, somatic approach that focuses on subtle processes, person-centered interventions, and post-traumatic growth. Aside from simply justification and a validation for this field that I dearly love and honor, the doctorate process and the writing of this book have allowed me to further elucidate upon the connection between the Expressive Therapies Continuum and the Neurosequential Model of Therapeutics and to advocate for and offer trauma interventions that give space for creativity, humor, joy, and reconnection to imagination.

I think that we are all waiting to know that there is something inside of us that can be drawn out, supported, and loved through the layers of shame and traumatic debris that may be present.

References

Gantt, L., & Tinnin, L. W. (2009). Support for a neurobiological view of trauma with implications for art therapy. *The Arts in Psychotherapy, 36,* 148–153. https://psycnet. apa.org/doi/10.1016/j.aip.2008.12.005

Klorer, P. G. (2005). Expressive therapy with severely maltreated children: Neuroscience contributions. *Art Therapy, 22*(4), 213–220. https://doi.org/10.1080/07421656 .2005.10129523

Robbins, T. (2003). *Skinny legs and all.* Bantam.

Talwar, S. (2007). Accessing traumatic memory through art making: An art therapy trauma protocol (ATTP). *The Arts in Psychotherapy, 34,* 22–35. https://psycnet.apa. org/doi/10.1016/j.aip.2006.09.001

Index